STUDIES OF CHILDREN

Monographs in Psychosocial Epidemiology

STUDIES OF CHILDREN

edited by Felton Earls

PRODIST
New York - 1980

First published in the United States by
PRODIST
a division of
Neale Watson Academic Publications, Inc.
156 Fifth Avenue, New York, NY 10010

"Longitudinal Methods for Research in Child Psychiatry"
by L. N. Robins is published courtesy Springer-Verlag, Heidelberg.

Library of Congress Cataloging in Publication Data

Main entry under title:

Studies of children.

(Monographs in psychosocial epidemiology; 1)
1. Child psychiatry—Research. 2. Child psychopathology—Research. 3. Epidemiology—Research. I. Earls, Felton. II. Series.
RJ500.2.S78 1980 618.92′89′0072 80-20158
ISBN 0-88202-132-X

Designed and manufactured in the U.S.A.

Table of Contents

Foreword

Rising costs of mental health care and interest in the development of a national health insurance that should include some mental health services have heightened concern for ways by which health planners may evaluate the extent of behavioral problems and the means by which the efficacy of various treatment modalities may be assessed. Questions of paramount importance include: If there exist two or more ways of treating an illness, which is the most effective? If two therapeutic modalities are equally effective, which is the most efficient? If equally efficient, which is the least costly? Questions regarding the prevalence and incidence rates of specific psychiatric illness in communities are being raised by those delegated with the task of making policy recommendations for programs of primary prevention and treatment. What is the natural history of a behavioral problem untreated and how is the problem affected by normal growth and development? What does a knowledge of the natural history of a disorder of mood, thought, or behavior tell us about its etiology, and how may it lead to methods of prevention? If an illness is not preventable by currently available knowledge, what interventions may be made in its natural history to arrest and possibly reverse its course? Mental health is now big business and failure to look at specific population needs when planning programs and to build in ways of evaluating cost-efficiency-effectiveness results in considerable psychological and economic cost to millions of patients and their families as well as taxpayers in general.

Epidemiology includes a number of technical skills used in answering some of the questions facing health planners today. Traditionally, epidemiology has been seen as the study of disease patterns in populations. Epidemiologists have provided data that have led to effective programs in the prevention of a number of infectious diseases including malaria, smallpox, and poliomyelitis. However, epidemiology has played a minor role in psychiatric research until relatively recently. Epidemiologic studies in mental health tended to be descriptive and focused on the prevalence and incidence rates of symptoms in broad diagnostic categories such as "neuroses" or "psychoses." In fact, some infectious and chronic disease epidemiologists question whether epidemiology can be used to tackle psychiatric problems. The Society for Epidemiologic Research does not have a section on psychosocial epidemiology, and the publication of papers in social and psychiatric epidemiology in the main journal of epidemiology is infrequent. The principal organs for the dispersion of knowledge in psychosocial epidemiology have been *Psychologi-*

cal Medicine and the *Archives of General Psychiatry*. The former journal, published quarterly, has on its editorial board members that are sophisticated in epidemiology, and probably publishes the greatest number of articles in this area. As a British journal it has limited readership in the United States. On the other hand, the *Archives of General Psychiatry,* a publication of the American Medical Association, is widely read in the United States. It publishes a number of high quality papers in epidemiology but has a broad mandate and, therefore, is limited in its ability to publish more.

The *Monograph Series in Psychosocial Epidemiology,* of which this is the premiere volume, is to serve several important functions for epidemiology, psychiatry, and related areas in public health. The objectives include:

1. Providing a forum for discussion of research strategies in the evaluation of mental health problems in the community and of assessing effectiveness of psychiatric treatment interventions;
2. Serving as a teaching tool for students in medical schools and schools of public health, hospital administration, social work, and nursing, as well as for students in departments of psychology and sociology and, especially, epidemiology;
3. Keeping prospective researchers alert to problems needing investigation in the area of psychosocial epidemiology;
4. Serving as a vehicle to bring together research in the area of psychosocial epidemiology;
5. Providing a means of continuing education for epidemiologists working in the field; and
6. Providing a means for discussions on how the results of epidemiologic and related behavioral research might be brought to bear on the development of state and federal health policy decisions.

To achieve these ends, each monograph will have a theme of particular interest to investigators in the field of psychosocial epidemiology such as the study of children, the study of stressful life events, and needs assessment. Each volume of the monograph will have a guest editor with an established reputation in the field chosen by us. The guest editor will direct the selection of the individual contributors and write the introductory article. In general, the lead article will: (1) contain a discussion of methodological considerations in the research of a given area (i.e., experimental design, sampling, instruments used, analysis of data, economic considerations and ethical decisions in planning studies), (2) critically review existing studies, (3) present information on the current state of the field, and (4) suggest directions for further research.

The volumes in the series, in addition to the present one on studying children epidemiologically, include ones on stressful life events, needs assessment, genetics, aging, alcohol use, ethics of epidemiologic research, drug use, community surveys, the methodology of natural experiments, and the interrelationships between psychological and physical responsiveness. Guest editors include Bruce P. and Barbara Snell Dohrenwend, Carl Eisdorfer, Stanislav V. Kasl, David Mechanic, Jerome Myers, Lee N. Robins, Marc Schuckett, Laurence R. Tancredi, Ming T. Tsuang, George Warheit, and Myrna M. Weissman. In addition to the introductory article and papers by selected investigators in the field, each issue will contain, whenever possible, an editorial written by a representative of the World Health Organization and by ourselves. The representative of WHO, chosen by Dr. Norman Sartorius, Director of the Division of Mental Health, will discuss what is being done internationally in the topic area; what should be done cooperatively and independently to advance the field; what WHO feels are research priorities in the field; and what particular methodological research problems exist in pretechnological and Third World nations. Our editorial will address the present state of epidemiological research in the area, the directions the Center for Epidemiological Studies at the National Institute of Mental Health would like to see research take, and the relationship of research in the field to the formulation of health policy.

The mandate of this series is challenging and the task great, but with the help of our guest editors and other contributors, and feedback from our readership, we can make the series special and sufficient to fulfill the need for an organ to draw together researchers, students, and health policy makers in an effort to reap from research in psychosocial epidemiology conclusions that lead to effective and consumer-responsive health policy and programs of preventive psychiatric care.

B. Z. L.
A. E. S.

Preface

High, and at times, number one in the priorities of the current and the previous Director of the National Institute of Mental Health has been emphasis on programs for children which include research and prevention. The priority given to children's needs has been further highlighted in the past year by its designation as the International Year of the Child and in the United States by the announcement of the Youth Initiatives in Alcoholism by the Secretary of Health, Education, and Welfare. Therefore, it seems fitting that the first in the *Monograph Series in Psychosocial Epidemiology* be devoted to children.

Despite the concern of the past decade and the amount of resources expended by NIMH, clearly we have, as the contributors to this volume attest, a long way to go. Programs of prevention are in need of development and still we are lacking evidence for the efficacy of the treatment of a number of psychological disorders of childhood. This is said not in discouragement nor is it meant to be discouraging. As stated in the report of the Ad Hoc Committee on Child Mental Health to the Director of the National Institute of Mental Health: "Knowledge tends to be achieved slowly and unpredictably out of the inspiration and energies of many investigators. 'Breakthroughs' rarely occur. What seems to the nonexpert to be a momentous, unheralded discovery is most often a small piece of knowledge that builds into many preceding, interlocking pieces after many discards and false tries" (1971, p. 27).

Felton Earls, the guest editor of this volume, states in the lead article that the purpose of his paper is to analyze the adaptation of epidemiologic methods and reasoning to child psychiatry. Epidemiologic research in child psychiatry is, however, as Achenbach points out later in the volume, handicapped by a lack of accepted diagnostic constructs and operational definitions. In addition, a major difficulty in the understanding of what is so-called normal and psychopathological behavior in children and the effects of a therapeutic intervention is a need to distinguish developmental influences on behavior from the real effects of therapy. When may we predict for a parent, for example, that a child will outgrow a behavior and when may we tell clinicians that a behavior is an indicant of psychopathology? Epidemiologic research can be of assistance in this matter and serves as a safeguard to broad generalizations of so-called "armchair psychiatrists." For many dynamically-oriented clinicians, turmoil in adolescence was once felt to be a normal concomitant of adolescence. Rutter's studies in England alluded to in

Earls's article, however, suggest this may not be so. It appears that turmoil is an exception, not a rule, and when present may be cause for concern. Longitudinal studies with samples of sufficient size which are representative of the populations from which they are chosen (and not just from one or more particular child psychoanalyst's files) are needed to help identify genetic, developmental, and environmental influences. In some cases of schizophrenia and alcoholism, genetic factors may be the dominant risk factors; in these instances we may not hope for prevention of adult dysfunction by early intervention. This should not negate the fact, however, Earls tells us that a child may require treatment for his-her own current needs even if not for prevention.

On a more optimistic note, we agree with Achenbach that epidemiologic research is not only possible without a total consensus on definitions but, in addition, it may be a needed step in formulating valid definitions. One major step in this direction stems from the success of the Epidemiologic Catchment Area Program recently initiated by the Division of Biometry and Epidemiology at NIMH. In developing the program aimed at determining specific mental disorders in the general populations aged 18 or older, a Diagnostic Interview Schedule (DIS) evolved from the work of previous investigators. The Division recently convened and is currently supporting several investigators interested in attempting to develop a diagnostic schedule suitable for populations younger than 18.

Recent emphasis on specific mental disorders as opposed to global measures of mental illness traditionally used, especially in child psychiatry, represents progress. Information on rates of specific disorders, Orvaschel, Sholomskas, and Weissman tell us in their paper, aids investigators in identification of risk factors, advances our knowledge of etiology, contributes to the determination of treatment needs, and provides a groundwork for preventive strategies. The lack of such information was quite explicit in the report of the President's Commission on Mental Health. For the development of programs of prevention based on an understanding of etiology rather than the vacillating interests of health care politicians, and to serve as a basis for reimbursement for treatment of childhood psychiatric disorders, a great deal of information will be needed. The identification of the fetal alcohol syndrome, for example, and the knowledge obtained regarding its etiology has been a major step in the prevention of yet another cause of childhood neurological impairment and of much pain to the parents of these children.

The Division of Biometry and Epidemiology recently contracted for a study of the role of pediatricians in the detection, treatment, and referral of patients with emotional, behavioral, and school problems. The Center for Epidemiologic Studies has begun work on evaluating the use of its depressive symptomatology scale (CES-D) with adolescents and young adults.

Through its grant program, the Center supports other research relevant to children which we cannot report in this monograph, due to limitation of space. This research includes: a longitudinal study of stress and related factors in the incidence of mental and behavioral problems among urban children originally in the 6- to 18-year-old range; research to develop screening methods for use with preschool children to determine the prevalence of behavioral, emotional, and cognitive dysfunction in 4-year-olds; and research evaluating the long-range effects of early hyperkinesis.

In response to the President's Commission on Mental Health, an Office of Prevention has recently been created in the National Institute of Mental Health. The thrust of the newly created office's activities has included a strong emphasis on programs related to children and youth. Its initial two major research grant initiatives both relate to this population. One is concerned with the impact of marital disruption (i.e., divorce/separation) on children, the other, with the impact of severely disturbed parents on children. More research needs to be done in this area aimed at the development of programs of primary, secondary, and tertiary prevention. We need to develop a greater empirical understanding of the real magnitude of factors commonly felt to play a serious role in the prevalence and incidence of adult psychopathology such as cultural and ethnic influences on child rearing and the early effects of varying social and economic conditions. The role may not be as great as one might expect nor should it necessarily be. Earls points out that we need additional information on the similarities and differences between populations and subpopulations in order to determine to what degree we may generalize findings from one area of the country or world to another. An understanding of generalizability of findings is necessary to develop needs assessment techniques similar to those of George Warheit's which may be used by health planners in community mental health centers with limited funds for their own research but a great need to obtain an understanding of what programs should be funded. Administrative epidemiology is the subspecialty of epidemiology that applies epidemiologic techniques to an understanding of cost-efficiency-effectiveness of therapeutic interventions and depends on findings from researchers in scientific epidemiology. Once knowledge of prevalence, incidence, and causality is elaborated, administrative epidemiologists seek to ascertain how a course of illness may be affected by programs of prevention and treatment. It seeks the answers to questions such as: Does psychotherapy in childhood have any significant role in the prevention of major adult psychopathology or does it serve principally to mollify the pain of a child and his or her parents?

Earls and the other contributors to this premiere volume of our monograph series provide an excellent overview of the key topics relevant both to scientific and to administrative epidemiologic studies of children. These include case definition, measurement development, and delineation of causal pathways. In addition, in this volume as in many future ones, special consideration will be given to legal and ethical issues such as informed consent, confidentiality, and the minimization of risk. Lee Robins's list of references provides the reader with a good sampling of productivity in the area of child epidemiology thus far.

In the main, the contributors to this monograph correctly emphasize the thorny conceptual and methodological thickets through which researchers must yet tread their way as they undertake epidemiologic studies of children. That such an endeavor is worthwhile is clear if you conclude as does Earls that in developing and in developed nations "*societies should be able to more effectively discharge the function of promoting the psychological health of children as an integral part of total health.*" To this end epidemiology *can* and *must* make a contribution. This volume is an effort in that direction.

B. Z. L.
A. E. S.

Epidemiologic Methods for Research in Child Psychiatry

FELTON EARLS, M.D.

Introduction

As epidemiology evolved from the study of the distribution and determinants of infectious diseases to an inquiry into various chronic diseases, some changes in concepts and tactics have been required (Terris, 1962). Much of the rethinking has been centered around the dimensions of time and duration of health disorders. Infectious disease epidemics are sudden in onset, sporadic in occurrence, and caused by factors which are relatively discrete in time and space. Chronic illnesses have insidious onsets, appear regularly in populations, and produce less clear evidence of a specific etiology. Since cholera, the plague, puerperal fever, and smallpox have been virtually eliminated from human populations, epidemiology has focused on the distribution and determinants of diseases of the circulatory system, cancer, accidents, and psychiatric morbidity. The origins of these chronic disorders is often difficult to pinpoint in time, and the threshold between premorbid states and clinically defined diseases is often based on arbitrary criteria.

The case of mental illness presents an intriguing situation in regard to its etiology and duration. The so-called "second revolution" in psychiatry presented a formidable body of theory suggesting that, at least, the nonpsychotic mental illnesses originated quite early in life (Freud, 1955). Though it is now clear that childhood experiences do not categorically give birth to adult psychiatric morbidity (Rutter, 1972), it must be admitted that much of the zeal that went into establishing the subdiscipline of child psychiatry at the beginning of the century had such a theory as its basis (Levy, 1968).

Children with emotional problems require treatment not for the sake of preventing adult psychiatric disorders, but because of their current needs. In this sense the revolutionary zeal of the mental hygiene movement was only partially unfounded. It is probably true that some types of nonpsychotic disorders, especially the most severe, do persist into adulthood (Robins, 1966). It may also be true that the major psychotic disorders, most of which become recognized clinically in adolescence and early adulthood, have important etiologic determinants in premorbid childhood experiences. This has become an increasingly less popular idea given an expanding body of evidence that these disorders have a genetic basis, but certainly the matter is far from conclusive (Kety et al., 1968). The epidemiologist interested in child psychiatric disorders or the child psychiatrist interested in epidemiologic methods is in the unique position of always being able to make two contributions with one effort, prevention of childhood disorder (primary, secondary, and tertiary) and the prevention of adult disorders (primary and secondary).

This chapter will analyze the adaptation of epidemiologic reasoning and methods to child psychiatry. Despite some singularly impressive studies which date back to the beginning of the mental hygiene movement, the history of epidemiologic efforts in child psychiatry is spotty (Earls, 1979). In the Americas such applications have lagged relative to developments in several European countries, most notably studies conducted in Great Britain (Graham, 1978). In the United States this is due in part to the ambiguous status of child psychiatry as a medical discipline: it has been aligned neither with pediatrics nor adult psychiatry, but instead has been more influenced by social work and the juvenile justice system.

A pre-epidemiologic phase in the history of child psychiatry can be recognized at a time when systematic inquiry was being applied to the study of behavior adjustment in aggregates of children with some consideration given to the population bases from which the samples were drawn. The studies of Wickman (1928), in which sources of observer bias (disagreement between teachers and psychiatrists) were analyzed; those of MacFarlane et al. (1954), in which developmental trends in behavior symptoms were charted; the pioneering surveys of Lewis (1929) on mental retardation; and the studies of Burt (1925), which examined the correlation of family and social patterns with juvenile delinquency—all are historical landmarks.

Over the past twenty years, epidemiology has been formally introduced into child psychiatry in such studies as those by La Pouse and Monk (1958) in America and Rutter (1970 a, b) in England. The concepts and methods used in these studies are reviewed and analyzed in this chapter. Germane to this discussion are two characteristics of the behavior of children which are implicit in any inquiry in child psychiatry or child development. These are the developmental trends in behavior and the dependent status of children. The first phenomenon requires that as a child matures biologically and socially, behavior reflects the maturation of neurophysiologic and neuropsychologic processes and acquires different interpersonal meaning for both the child and his caretaker. Secondly, the lengthy period of physical and emotional development required for the human species to reach full maturity carries with it risks and vulnerabilities toward a wide range of environmental effects. The origins and course of childhood psychiatric disorders, pitted against a background of developmental trends, are complex processes requiring the most persistent and diligent scientific efforts imaginable. Epidemiologic contributions to this endeavor are indispensable to this objective.

Eight methodological issues are discussed: (1) case definition, (2) sampling, (3) construction of hypothesis, (4) measurement, (5) types of epidemiologic studies, (6) research designs, (7) development of causal pathways, and (8) ethical and legal principles guiding epidemiologic research. Having reached the point at which preparation of such a review is useful in itself suggests that child psychiatry and epidemiology have progressed sufficiently to have developed an enduring collaborative link. It is hoped that this review will stimulate the kind of critical appraisal between these two fields that will sustain the momentum already established.

Domains of Psychiatric Epidemiology

Psychiatric epidemiology may be divided into two major branches, both concerned with ways of thinking about and examining mental health phenomena in large groups living under natural circumstances. Scientific epidemiology is primarily directed toward understanding causes, while administrative epidemiology applies to questions regarding health planning and the design and utilization of services. Administrative epidemiology and evaluation research, two related activities, are of great significance in themselves but are not related to unraveling the causes of psychiatric disorders. The search for the biological, social, and cultural causes of child psychiatric disorders is in the more classical tradition of epidemiology. While epidemiologic approaches of this sort may have a contribution to make to administrative needs, these two domains of epidemiology are sufficiently different to warrant independent analyses. The emphasis in this chapter is on etiologically directed epidemiology. Considering the vast number of questions unanswered and the rather spotty history of epidemiology in child psychiatry, this level of restriction may prove beneficial.

Definition of Key Terms

Before considering the variety of epidemiologic studies and their limitations, it is useful to define a few key terms. The selection of terms is by no means exhaustive, but instead is chosen to help clarify the unique contributions that epidemiology may make to child psychiatry research.

A *case* is a person designated to have a psychiatric disorder or to carry a substantial risk of developing one.

Prevalence is defined as the number of cases existing in a population at a given moment or period in time. Prevalence studies require a definition of disorder, a method of measuring the disorder under question, and a knowledge of the population base from which the sample is taken. Prevalence may be estimated by the application of a variety of abbreviated techniques, such as a screening questionnaire or a shortened physical examination. True prevalence, however, is taken as a more reliable index and is typically based on adjustment of an estimated prevalence by applying more extensive examination to the population at risk or mathematically, by applying a correction term to the estimated prevalence based on the known sensitivity and specificity of the screening method used (Rogan, 1978). Occasionally the word prevalence refers to treated prevalence. This is an inappropriate use of the term if demographic characteristics of the population base from which the sample was taken and the variety of factors influencing how children as patients ultimately got to treatment facilities are unknown.

Incidence refers to the number of new cases defined in the population over a given interval of time. The incidence of behavior disorder may be obtained if the prevalence and duration are known by applying the formula:

$$P = I \times D$$

where P is prevalence, I is incidence, and D is duration. Prevalence studies frequently disregard the types of behavior disorders occurring in a population, particularly if they are being used for administrative purposes. Incidence studies must specify the types of disorders under consideration since their durations may be quite different. A variety of other concerns to be discussed in subsequent sections of this chapter make incidence studies more demanding scientifically than prevalence studies.

The remaining definitions have to do with the ways in which associations between cause and effect are drawn in epidemiologic investigations. If the dependent variable is established as a satisfactory measure of the disorder in question, a variety of independent variables may be associated with it, and the strength of the association may be tested statistically. Since the majority of epidemiologic studies explain associations on a causal basis, a customary means of expressing the relationship between independent and dependent variables is known as *relative risk*. This index compares the rate of occurrence of a presumed causal factor in subjects possessing both the factor and the disorder with subjects in whom the factor exists in the absence of the disorder. Since relative risk is routinely used in retrospective studies (though it may be used in prospective studies as well), the meaning of the association established must be regarded cautiously in causal terms. A number of statistical techniques, such as path analysis (Wright, 1978), have been established to permit powerful analyses of patterns of association when many independent variables are taken into account.

Since all psychiatric disorders require time to develop and involve the interaction of a host of influences, a useful contribution of epidemiologic methodology is the concept of *causal chain*. A causal chain is a specific ordering of independent variables arranged sequentially in time which eventually produce a mental disorder. The chain may be divided into *proximal factors* and *distal factors* to denote their influence over time. Mediating variables may also be inserted in the chain to alter a person's susceptibility to developing the disorder. If the ordering of variables in the chain is highly specific, then a substantial reordering of factors should fail to bring about the designated mental disorder. For example, if the combination of variables—perinatal stress, physical abuse, school failure, and membership in a delinquent subculture—are considered a causal chain leading to antisocial personality disorder, then it is necessary to assume that all four factors must be present in a fixed sequence. This is like describing necessary and sufficient conditions in the construction of hypotheses.

In specifying a causal chain, variables may be categorized in a number of ways to fit the investigator's particular research questions. In examining the etiology of schizophrenia, for example, a causal chain might include genetic, intrafamilial, and extrafamilial factors. Further, variables in a causal chain may be specified in terms of developmental trends and events. For example, reading failure in the first three or four years of school might be a necessary condition for the development of adolescent delinquency. The timing of this event is specific, and when added to other conditions occurring at earlier and later points in development, it becomes part of a set of sufficient conditions. A wide range of factors may operate at specific developmental epochs to increase the vulnerability of the child to develop a psychiatric disorder, provided it is followed by other specific events. Sameroff and Chandler (1975) have developed this concept in developmental theory and use the expression "transaction" rather than causal chain to describe the time-dependent linkage of events.

The distinction between proximal and distal factors might also be conceived in terms of *onset conditions* and *etiologic factors*. Etiologic factors refer to those which are fundamental to the development of a particular disorder such as genetic factors in schizophrenia or brain dysfunction in hyperkinesis. Onset conditions are thought to be fundamentally responsible for precipitating the appearance of a disorder. A plausible case has been made for the role of stressful life events in determining the time of onset of depressive illnesses in women (Brown and Harris, 1978). The distinction is important, since the two are frequently blurred in causal thinking. An important function of theories and model building in epidemiologic research is to reconstruct the circumstances and events in a child's life which give rise to psychiatric disorders. The particular power of the epidemiologic approach is that it can test a causal chain empirically in a broad population base. Theory and empirically based findings can then be integrated to refine a hypothetical causal chain. This may be done by ordering the variables more specifically, deleting some, or by adding a greater number of mediating variables.

Case Definition

As Mechanic (1970) pointed out, the strength of any epidemiologic study is based on the accuracy of its dependent variable. In most studies the dependent variable is a behavioral characteristic or group of characteristics, the definition of which represents either an established or incipient psychiatric disorder.

Two fundamental problems arise in case definition. The first is based on decisions regarding the limits and range of behavior problems that may constitute a psychiatric disorder. For child psychiatrists this is a function not only of the type of behavior being examined but also of the age and maturity of the child. The symptom of stereotyped movements may be classed as deviant behavior at almost any age but is not assumed to contribute to psychiatric disorder unless it occurs in a context of other deviant behaviors. The clinical salience of such a symptom is a function of age and the nature of associated behaviors. When associated with an absence of speech in a child over the age of thirty months, a diagnosis of infantile autism is strongly indicated. In a child less than this age and without the same associated behaviors, the same characteristic may represent a different syndrome with a distinct etiology and prognosis. Progress is being made in classification and diagnosis of child psychiatric disorders, but much important work remains before the limits of these disorders are thoroughly described in terms of developmental trends and the clustering of behavioral characteristics in the form of syndromes (Rutter, 1975a).

Some disorders such as the personality disorders are conveniently thought to exist on a continuum ranging from normal to deviant, while disorders such as childhood schizophrenia have little overlap with normal behavioral adaptations. Some disorders are defined on the basis of single items of behavior such as enuresis, tics, encopresis, or hair-pulling, while still others require several characteristics of behavior to coexist within the same person for proper delineation. This range of definitions confronts the epidemiologist interested in characterizing the various types of childhood psychiatric disorders.

A second problem in case definition relates to the orientation and perceived applicability of an investigation. Epidemiologic research in psychiatry typically has assumed either a clinical or statistical approach to diagnosis and classification. Clinically oriented studies assume that undeclared cases of psychiatric disorder existing in the general population are broadly similar to declared cases in a clinic population (Ingham and Miller, 1976). In fact, clinically oriented studies have routinely defined the validity of case identification techniques by their capacity to discriminate true cases from matched controls (Wing et al., 1978). For example, in the Isle of Wight study a series of reliability and validity studies based on the capacity of parent and child interview methods to select cases (children attending a psychiatric facility) from controls (children matched on all pertinent characteristics except for the fact that they were not attending a psychiatric clinic) preceded application of this technique to a general population (Graham and Rutter, 1968; Rutter and Graham, 1968). While there is contradictory evidence that there exists, at least for emotional disorders of childhood, a fundamental difference between declared and undeclared cases (Shepherd et al., 1966), the reasoning implied in the clinical approach carries with it the danger of circularity.

Sociologically oriented studies typically abandon clinical definitions at the outset of an epidemiologic investigation, either by arbitrarily defining a certain threshold above which certain behavioral characteristics are defined as a disorder or by carrying out statistical procedures such as factor and cluster analyses to define syndromes. The definition of disorder in these studies is arrived at as a *result* of carrying out a survey in a nonclinical population and not on *a priori* assumptions of what constitutes a psychiatric disorder. Often an investigation will have elements of both approaches. La Pouse's pioneering work serves as an illustration of how case definition can be expanded in the context of an evolving analysis of behavior problems from a population perspective. Beginning with definitions based on single symptoms, such as fears or worries (La Pouse and Monk, 1959), a more elaborate and clinically meaningful definition was reached by including a wider range of social adjustment characteristics in a statistically based definition (La Pouse and Monk, 1965).

A major development in child psychiatry case definition was the demonstration by Glidewell et al. (1957) that a symptom-loading approach to diagnosis provides a practical method of identifying large groups of children with psychiatric disorder. The method is now commonly used in a variety of behavior scales for children (Rutter, 1967; Conners, 1969). Most recently, this technique has been developed by Richman and Graham (1971) for the identification of behavior problems in 3-year-old children. In their epidemiologic study it was shown that the number of symptoms a child had agreed well with ratings made from a clinical perspective (Richman et al., 1975).

Despite the progress being made, an uncomfortable degree of disparity remains in current work. Review of three of the largest and most influential epidemiologic studies completed in child psychiatry over the last ten years point out such differences. Kellam et al.'s (1975) study of first graders relies heavily on teacher ratings of social adaptation and the children's own subjective ratings of psychological well-being. Definitions of disorder are extracted from the distribution of scores on both these methods. Rutter et al.'s (1970a) work combines parents' and teachers' questionnaires and interviews, and children's interviews, but such small degrees of overlap between these three domains require that case identification be made only if a child has high scores on at least two of the three techniques. Finally, the New York based work by Langner et al. (1974), which is the most sociological of the three, is based on parent report techniques supplemented by official records. It relies heavily on multivariate statistical approaches to define types of behavioral syndromes existing in a general population (Eisenberg et al., 1976). Some of the syndromes derived in this fashion have quite clear clinical salience, whereas others do not.

There are few published accounts of investigations which attempt to replicate and refine existing techniques in populations different from ones for which the techniques were originally developed. Rutter's (1967) teacher questionnaire has been used in a sample of Italian school children (Zimmerman-Tansella et al., 1978), and Earls (1980a) used a parent questionnaire designed and used in Great Britain in an American study. Such cross-national attempts at replicating results with the same method represent an essential means of assessing the extent to which features of children's behavior disorders are universal.

Depending on the purpose and type of study, case definition may be limited to the clustering of symptoms, or to a more inclusive (i.e., multiaxial) approach to defining psychiatric phenomena. The former approach is limited to screening inventories, some of which are designed to detect specific disorders such as autism, while others are nonspecific. If relevant biological and social factors are to be included in the definition, lengthy interviews or repeated interviews are necessary.

Sampling

Sampling procedures in child psychiatry research involve at least four separate considerations: sample size, representativeness, generalizability, and population stability. In approaching the question of sample size, the researcher is faced with making estimates on the frequency of occurrence of certain select variables in a population of interest. It may not be immediately obvious that a sample of 100, 500, or 2,000 is required to make definitive results. Furthermore, there is a constraint on staff size, time, and money. Therefore, one wants a sufficiently large sample to carry out a complete analysis, but not so large that inordinate amounts of time and money are spent in data collection.

In general, studies which employ face-to-face interviewing are more time consuming and expensive than those which rely on self-report or paper-and-pencil methods. If the intention is to conduct a multistaged investigation, the size of sample initially involved will have to be large enough to generate sufficient numbers in the subsequent stages for analysis. All these considerations warrant that the investigator has some evidence of what to expect from a particular population. Such evidence may be obtained from public records containing demographic characteristics of population groups. For example, it might be expected that urban populations will have a higher proportion of psychiatrically impaired children than rural areas, or that areas reporting high crime rates within an urban area will have high rates of delinquency as well as other types of psychiatric disorders (Cooper and Gath, 1977). But ultimately, the investigator will want to go beyond these kinds of qualitative guesses to a means of making a quantitive estimate of the sample size required. Since the investigator will have defined a dependent variable and obtained one or more methods of measuring it at the first stage of planning an investigation, knowledge on how these dependent variables have behaved in previous studies is most useful.

Techniques used in previous studies are helpful to the investigation since they may serve as a basis for estimating the sample size required to conduct a new study. Even if the measure has only been used in a clinical context, knowledge of its standard error can serve as a basis for estimating sample size. In this case the formulas used (Barker and Rose, 1976) are:

$$(1)\ \ SE = \sqrt{\frac{P(100 - P)}{n}}$$

SE = Standard error
P = Prevalence
n = Sample size

$$(2)\ \ SEM = \sqrt{\frac{s^2}{n}}$$

SEM = Standard error of the mean
s = Subject standard deviation
n = Sample size

The first formula is based on the standard error of a proportion and is used to estimate random sampling error in a prevalence study, that is, the extent to which a sample may be unrepresentative of the population from which it was drawn. Once the investigator has decided how precisely he wishes to measure a crucial variable (determined by the SE) and what the approximate frequency of the condition is in the population (P), the equation may be solved for the required sample size (n). For example, for a condition with an estimated prevalence of 10 percent, a sample size of 225 is needed to assure the investigator that the sample estimate of the prevalence has a 95 percent chance of being within two standard errors of the true population value.

The second formula is used for variables assumed to be continuously distributed in a population. Many behavior scales used in psychiatry research are based on this assumption. If an estimate of the standard error of the mean of the measure to be used and an estimate of between-subject variability are known, the sample size can be calculated.

While these formulas are most useful in setting the lower limits for sample size, they may also be helpful in showing upper limits beyond which an increase in number results in negligible gains in the precision of measurement. Of course, vastly different sample sizes are needed for conditions of relatively low prevalence (where the frequency may be less than 1 per 1,000) and personality disorders (Barker and Rose, 1976).

Another method in estimating sample size is to prepare one or more final crucial tables, once a set of variables and a research design are decided upon. Preparation of such "mock-up" tables allows one to insert estimated cell sizes based on the best information available.

In case-control studies the selection of a control group through a method of matching is required. The purpose of matching is to achieve two groups which differ only according to the crucial variables of immediate interest. This is usually a most difficult exercise in the social sciences because of the many confounding variables that may influence an outcome. Proper matching involves planning a strategy at the beginning of a study that insures group comparability. This may be done through paired sampling, such as the sampling frame of a school district, whose experimental and control children may be chosen from the same classroom. All too often the control group and the selection of variables to be controlled are rapidly assembled after the experimental group has already been established. This results in a rather unbalanced state of affairs in which more attention has been given to selection of cases than to the control group. This leads to considerable difficulties. An example is that most or all of the control group may be interviewed after the experimental group, leading to systematic biases arising from changes in interviewing skill or content. Another pitfall of matching involves the careful selection of confounding variables to be controlled. It is often tempting to match on too many variables, a situation which can make it impossible to find a suitable number of controls for complete comparison (McMahon and Pugh, 1970).

Considerable pain is taken in epidemiology to arrive at a representative sample. Representativeness is usually defined in terms of a general population. To achieve a representative sample of a general population, either random or systematic sampling techniques are used. Both require a means of enumerating all persons in the population (e.g., through a birth register). Random samples employ a probability scheme to insure that as each person is selected, all remaining subjects have an equal opportunity of being selected on the next round. Systematic samples employ a fixed format to draw names from a file or register (e.g., a one-in-four sample). Of the two the random sample is safer since it avoids any chance that the particular format adopted in the systematic approach accidentally strikes at some inherent property of the list itself. The only rationale for choosing a systematic approach to sampling is its convenience, since considerable problems may arise in insuring that randomization and representativeness are being preserved when one is sampling large numbers. Despite the additional effort, random samples remain the most valid evidence that representativeness has been achieved.

To achieve balance on a variable of particular concern in a sample, stratification may be included in the sampling technique. This gives some assurance that sufficient numbers will be obtained among important categories. It is frequently desirable to stratify a sample by social class, race, neighborhood, census tracts, or other demographic variables. Of course, the list from which names are drawn must indicate levels of the variable to be stratified.

The power of any epidemiologic study is the degree to which its findings can be generalized to other groups. It is common to base such estimates of generalizability on demographic characteristics, child-rearing methods, or other such variables. However, an impressive case can be made for the possibility that the kinds of social factors causing child psychiatric disorder vary more in quantity than in quality from population to population. Rutter found that similar factors were linked to psychiatric disorder in children living in inner-London and the Isle of Wight (Rutter et al., 1975b). In 3-year-olds, Earls and Richman (1980b, 1980c) failed to find differences in the frequency of behavior problems in children from West Indian families and indigenous families living in an outer London borough, despite differences in social and cultural factors. Even more impressive is the similarity in prevalence between the children living in London and those living in an American rural community (Earls, 1980a).

The estimation of total prevalence is quite a superficial measure. A 10% prevalence in one population may not be composed of the same kinds or severity of disturbances found in another group, and their causes may be different. Studies of incidence and in-depth case analyses are necessary to further define the similarities and differences between populations or subpopulations.

Until more is known, it would be wise to base the limits of generalizability on demographic markers. For example, Earls (1980a) conservatively describes the limits of generalizability of an epidemiologic study on Martha's Vineyard island to rural Atlantic seacoast settings which economically depend on seasonal tourism as a main industry. Even such a restricted degree of generalizability substantially increases the number of children to which findings of this study might be extended, as there are many similar communities. Less conservatively, the limits of generalizability in this study extend to all 3-year-olds living in American rural communities. It might even be argued that the findings of this study could be extended to all American families with 3-year-old children, since the conditions giving rise to some types of behavior problems are primarily intrafamilial (Robins, 1978). However, this results in the kind of overstatement which the epidemiologist should guard against. Political, social or economic structure, cultural and ethnic influences on child rearing, geographic and demographic factors—all are factors commonly thought to have some influence on prevalence and incidence, though they need not necessarily be as large as one might suspect.

Finally, some mention should be made of population stability. Since studies on children are inherently of a developmental nature, it is imperative to contemplate follow-up and longitudinal designs. Indexes of in-migration and out-migration are difficult to assess even in small, demarcated communities. Yet, some indexes may be available, e.g., annual voter registration lists, school rosters, and the number of high school graduates leaving a community. In planning a study, efforts should be made to investigate such information periodically, since population stability may be subject to rapid historical changes, particularly in American society.

Hypothesis Generation and Hypothesis Testing

Few studies in epidemiologic child psychiatry have stated a hypothesis and then proceeded through a series of investigations to confirm or disconfirm what was originally postulated. This is in part due to the fact that epidemiology is not a laboratory science. Experimentation in epidemiology generally involves seizing naturally occurring events or public records, and then convincing large numbers of persons to give time to discuss matters which might otherwise remain their private concerns. These features of epidemiologic research represent enormous problems in themselves, often requiring a major effort on the part of investigators just to get a study started. Many compromises are usually made from the time an idea for a study is first entertained until actual data collection commences. During this interval an explicit statement of a hypothesis may appear less important to the investigator than securing the study.

Another reason for the dearth of hypothesis testing is a lack of confidence in the quality of measurement, especially that regarding the definitions of disorders. Major efforts are currently under way to define psychiatric disorders more precisely and to gain knowledge on their etiology and natural history (Rutter et al., 1975a; American Psychiatric Association, 1978). These pursuits will have a positive influence toward developing a scientifically robust child psychiatry.

Given the present level of development in child psychiatry, there are several ways of generating hypotheses using epidemiologic approaches:

1. By comparing populations or subpopulations to examine historical, economic, cultural, or biological differences;
2. By examining the association of various factors with recognized disorder;
3. By charting developmental trends; and
4. By predicting outcomes.

Any particular epidemiologic study will probably have a major investment in one of the above areas. The quality of the investigation will be enhanced if time is given to spelling out the underlying assumptions at its beginning. Even if specific hypotheses are not formally stated, the process of creating them is improved by tackling assumptions at the outset of an investigation. Indeed, the generation and refinement of hypotheses is a never-ending process of reworking one's assumptions. Some large-scale surveys have been conducted with no more of an objective than finding the frequency of a condition in a population. This is not the work of a science and should not be misconstrued as such. Epidemiologic science requires a process of making explicit the theories, the assumptions, and the propositions guiding an investigation.

Quality of Measurement

Two considerations guide an understanding of the quality and limitations of measurement in child psychiatry: the nature of variables used, and sources and types of error expected. Variables are created by imparting categorical distinctions to phenomena of interest to the investigator. The categories are then assigned numbers, defining a range of expected variation. Depending on the properties tapped by the categorical distinctions made, a level of measurement is assigned to the variable. This level of measurement exists as a logical framework for classifying the assumptions an investigator is willing to make when comparing subjects or attributes of subjects. Of the four levels of measurement used—ratio, interval, ordinal, and nominal—epidemiologic studies rely heavily on ordinal scales. Ratio and interval scales permit inferences about the distance between categories or points in a scale, while ordinal scales permit only an ordering of categories along the same axis without allowing assumptions on the distance between points making up the scale. Unfortunately, many of the advanced statistical techniques routinely used in the social sciences are based on the assumption that variables be defined in terms of interval or ratio scales. It has become a convention to apply these techniques to situations in which measurement has been on an ordinal scale and to justify the exception by stating that the statistical procedures are robust.

Once a framework for measuring variables is made, a further classification of variables into independent and dependent status is made. This is based on the function that the variable is assigned in the research design. Independent variables are those which are designed to predict or explain some effect or response in the dependent variables. The dependent variables are typically synonymous with case definition. The same variable may also serve different functions depending on the series of questions pursued.

The sources and types of error expected in measurement command much of the investigator's time and commitment. These are the matters of validity and reliability, which are illustrated schematically in fig. 1. Validity is the more strategic concept to tackle in child psychiatric research, since behavior is a complex, multiply determined, and unstable entity to measure. Focusing mainly on behavior disorders, as is traditional in child psychiatry, may sim-

FIGURE 1

Components of the Quality of Measurement

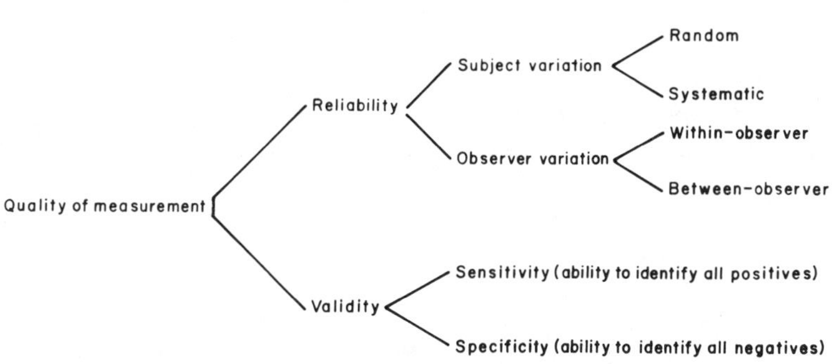

plify the matter to some extent if one is interested primarily in one tail of a distribution of complex behavioral attributes. In an area where normality and abnormality are largely coextensive, such narrowing of scope is inappropriate. Indeed, the broader scope on the range of normality and abnormality represents an essential contribution of epidemiologic approaches in this field (Leighton, 1979).

Behavior disorders are influenced, if not determined by, developmental trends; physiological states; family, school, and community settings; and parent and teacher perceptions. Therefore, the capacity of any method to measure behavior disorders is largely determined by the extent to which it responds to these issues. A parent questionnaire must be shown to deal with the problem of expectable biases in parent reports (Ferguson et al., 1974). This conceivably can be handled in a number of ways: by making observations of the behavior reported by the parents (remembering to keep contextual variables and developmental age constant), by comparing parent reports with an independent clinical assessment of the child, or by determining how well the parent report differentiates children already declared to be cases from those not so declared (Richman and Graham, 1971).

Each of the three types of validating procedures has its own imperfections. For the observational comparison, the investigator must know how to insure that the observations are conducted under the same conditions as the parents observed them in their natural setting. The investigator must know, or at least be able to estimate, what effect the observer's presence acts as an artifact on the child's behavioral output (Hughes et al., 1979). A clinically oriented assessment opens the way for theoretical or experiential biases on the part of the clinicians in interpreting data. In this sense it might be interesting to compare pediatricians with child psychiatrists in making judgments on behavior disorders in children, based on the assumption that the clinical experience of the pediatrician might yield a bias toward perceiving deviant behavior as normal. On the other hand, the child psychiatrist might be expected to have a bias toward interpreting normal behavior as deviant. Finally, allowing the determination of validity to rest on the capacity to discriminate between children attending or not attending a psychiatric facility opens the way to all the biases attendant on how children eventually reach a psychiatric service in the first place (Shepherd et al., 1966). For example, a parent questionnaire may be biased toward perceptual artifacts which obscure the emotional status of the child. At the same time parent-child interactional factors may be quite crucial in determining the parent's desire to seek intervention. In using such a biased questionnaire, the investigator is protected only to the extent that the behavior disorder he is attempting to validate is highly correlated with parent-child interaction.

Another way of expressing validity derived from epidemiology is in terms of sensitivity and specificity. Sensitivity is the capacity of a measure to select persons who actually have the disorder which is being measured. Therefore, it is an expression of the proportion of true cases out of all possible true cases selected by a particular measure. Specificity is an expression of the capacity of a measure to select persons who are truly free of the disorder. Formulas for sensitivity and specificity, along with four other commonly employed expressions of validity, are shown in table 1, using data from a total population survey of 3-year-old children (Earls, 1980a). The table presents findings at three different thresholds on the distribution of scores from a screening instrument and demonstrates how accuracy is a function of selecting different thresholds.

Several concepts of validity are used in psychological research including: convergent, discriminant, predictive, content, concurrent, and ecological. While each of these types has a significant function in understanding the separate components of validity, it is important not to become sidetracked by the unwieldy demands of satisfying each type. The critical issue in validity from an epidemiologic

TABLE 1

MEASUREMENT CHARACTERISTICS OF THE BEHAVIOR SCREENING QUESTIONNAIRE AT THREE THRESHOLD LEVELS

(in Percentages)

Characteristic	Formula	T 1 (BSQ=8)	T 2 (BSQ=10)	T 3 (BSQ=11)
Sensitivity	$\frac{TP}{TP+FN}$	100	78	64
Specificity	$\frac{TN}{TN+FP}$	70	85	98
Predictive Value Positive	$\frac{TP}{TP+FP}$	35	46	82
Predictive Value Negative	$\frac{TN}{TN+FN}$	100	96	94
False Positive Rate	$\frac{FP}{TN+FP}$	30	15	2
False Negative Rate	$\frac{FN}{TP+FN}$	0	12	36

TP=True Positive FP=False Positive
TN=True Negative FN=False Negative

perspective is to ensure that a measure used for one purpose (e.g., screening) is compared with another type of measure assumed to represent a more clinically or statistically robust reflection of the true condition under investigation. The one measure should be independent of the other.

While validity is synonymous with accuracy in measurement, reliability is the same as precision. It is impossible to have satisfactory validity without reliability, but the more unfortunate circumstance is to have a reliable measure which is not valid. Two types of reliability usually reported are the agreement between more than one observer or rater (interrater reliability) and the stability of measure over time (reproducibility, repeatability, or test-retest reliability). In addition to simple measures of percentage agreement between raters, a variety of formulas for reliability coefficients are available (Shrout and Fleiss, 1979). Depending on the particular formula used, minimized or maximized levels of agreement are obtained. Figure 2 illustrates the range of possible combinations of validity and reliability.

One of the advantages of epidemiologic studies which are based on large samples is the reduction of random subject error (see fig. 1). Both subject-related and observer-related sources of systematic variation exist. Many sources of subject bias such as age, sex, and social class are known; and if not controlled in the research design, at least their potential to reduce reliability can be acknowledged. Much of the pretesting, quality control, and standardization of procedure in an epidemiologic study is aimed at achieving and maintaining a high level of reliability between raters. Through

FIGURE 2

Schematic Representation of the Relationships Between Reliability and Validity

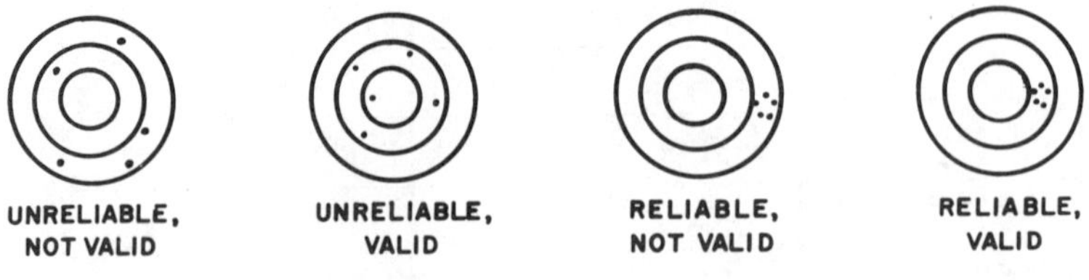

High validity is represented by dots approximating the center of the target, and high reliability, by dots which cluster together.

training, the investigator has a measure of control over reliability, but not much can be done about validity once a measure is employed. It is wise, therefore, to select measures on the basis of preestablished validity.

As a final point, epidemiologists should consult often with laboratory psychologists and clinicians about the development of new techniques for demonstrating validity and improving reliability. The multitrait, multimethod approach to validity described by Campbell and Fiske (1959) is a case in point. This approach represents a way to compensate for the variety of sources of error in measuring behavior using several different methods.

The evaluation of the reliability and validity of techniques available to investigators interested in child development is not a very serviceable task. Few methods have been the subject of carefully conducted studies on the quality of measurement techniques, and those which have been often suggest room for significant improvements. A recently published developmental assessment scale for neonates is an example of a technique reportedly high in reliability but considered low in validity (Als et al., 1977). The scale is fairly simple in design, and observers may be readily trained to reach a high level of interrater reliability in administering the scale. These features could make it attractive to the epidemiologist. For example, in a prospective study to examine the relationship of infant behavior to later cognitive, neurological, or behavioral development, this scale could serve as an initial measure of the infant's developmental status. Fortunately, an extensive review of this scale is available so that its selection can be made on rational grounds (Sameroff, 1979). However, few behavioral or developmental assessment techniques have been subjected to such an exhaustive review.

All too frequently in child psychiatric research, the investigator fails to find a satisfactory behavior scale, interview technique, or observational technique. This, then, evokes the need to invent a new technique, often by integrating fragments of other unsatisfactory methods. This is an undesirable ploy, particularly for epidemiologic studies, because it necessitates that the investigator demonstrate a reasonable level of validity and reliability of the new method before using it in a large-scale study. Unless the epidemiologist is particularly interested in designing new techniques, this activity can prove to be quite formidable, serving to sidetrack the investigator. Perhaps the wisest advice to the epidemiologist selecting measures for a new study is Whitehead's dictum on science: "Seek simplicity and distrust it."

Types of Studies and Research Designs

Several types of studies represent the epidemiologic approach. Rather than epidemiology connoting a particular type of study, it designates a particular rationale, a heuristic basis for pursuing knowledge on the distribution and determinants of psychiatric disorders in known population groups. It is common to think of epidemiology as limited to studies on the prevalence of disorders. While this is a cornerstone of epidemiology because it immediately places a particular disorder in a population perspective, epidemiologic studies may use case-control designs, natural history approaches, longitudinal or cohort designs, and clinical or field trials. This section considers these various types of studies.

Prevalence studies are of interest because of their potential for both the scientific and administrative applications. They may be limited either to a narrow age period or to a broad spectrum of ages. When applied to a spectrum of ages, they are termed cross-sectional studies. Prevalence studies are important in demonstrating that brief diagnostic procedures are useful in screening large populations. Once the accuracy of a screening technique is found satisfactory, it can be used to compare populations of different national, cultural, or demographic characteristics. Prevalence studies are also important in beginning the process of hypothesis generation. In fact, it may be the first attempt to extend a clinically derived hypothesis to a population base.

Because preparation for a large-scale prevalence study is a formidable task in itself, investigators often feel the urge to include a great number of categories of variables in the data collection procedure. This commonly results in exploratory data analyses which attempt through a variety of statistical techniques to discover patterns of association which are meaningful. Of course, this is done because interview time is precious. An abundance of information is often obtained in well-conducted prevalence studies. Nevertheless, the prevalence study may be quite limited in its scientific utility, because it cannot establish causal relationships, onset conditions, or the duration of disorders. Such studies, at their best, give only a static picture of emotional disorders. Given the dynamic processes of child development, this is an important limitation and is probably a primary reason why many investigators consider it mandatory to follow a sample over time.

Studies on the incidence of psychiatric disorder are inherently of greater scientific interest to the epidemiologist because causal hypotheses may be tested. Few studies in epidemiologic child psychiatry have explored this important type of study, but some longitudinal studies have attempted to make estimates on incidence (Chazan and Jackson, 1971, 1976).

The major difficulty in studies of incidence is defining the onset of disorder. Testing causal hypotheses is ideally done by closely approximating in time the presumed causal factor with the onset of disturbed behavior, but this is difficult in child psychiatry due to the complexity and subtleness which separates normal from abnormal behavior in the evolution of psychiatric disorders. It is typical to use contact with a service as the definition of onset, but this may be quite inappropriate since factors influencing contact with a service may obscure more naturally occurring behavior. To date, the question of how to date the onset of psychiatric disorders is largely unexplored, and the duration of disorders is largely unknown.

Factors influencing duration are also largely unknown. Most cross-sectional studies on prevalence do not report vast differences in the frequency of behavior difficulty with age. Typically, younger children are reported to have higher prevalences (MacFarlane, 1954; La Pouse and Monk, 1964; Langner, 1974). This might be interpreted to mean that as development proceeds, abnormal behavior becomes more readily discernible from normal behavior so that false positives are removed from the estimate of prevalence. But there is, in fact, insufficient information on duration of child psychiatric disorders from an epidemiologic perspective, except for antisocial personality disorders (Robins, 1978; Gersten et al., 1976). Rutter et al. (1976) have suggested that disorders having their first appearance in adolescence are not associated with the same constellation of family factors as those with an earlier onset and that the sex ratio tends to be more nearly balanced in adolescence. Further work is needed, however, to substantiate these findings.

Prevalence and incidence studies can, of course, generate their own case-control research designs when the population bases are broad, but case-control studies might also be the primary focus of an epidemiologic study. An example is Shepherd's study of a child guidance clinic population (Shepherd et al., 1966). In this study children attending the clinic were compared with a control group of children from the same community on a variety of behavioral, parental, and demographic characteristics. Findings from this study suggest that children attending the clinic were not distinguished by their disturbed behavior as much as they were by parental factors.

Of the several research designs used by epidemiologists, the controlled clinical trial is the most definitive. Longitudinal and incidence studies may give evidence that a particular association of independent and dependent variables is real, and not spurious. They may even suggest that a particular causal variable accounts for a high proportion of variance in the dependent variable. The clinical trial, however, confirms or disconfirms once and for all the extent to which the causal variable actually influences the presence and characteristics of a particular disorder. Again there are few examples of clinical trials in epidemiologic child psychiatry. Clinical trials are applied most typically in clinical settings to evaluate treatment approaches, but as a field trial they may also be applied to preventive measures in child psychiatry such as the one conducted by Cullen (1976).

Research designs used by epidemiologists may also be categorized as longitudinal or cross-sectional. Longitudinal studies examine the effect of independent variables on dependent variables at two or more points in time. They may be either prospective or retrospective in design. A prospective longitudinal study is one in which data on explanatory variables is collected prior to data collection on the response variables. In a retrospective longitudinal study, data on the explanatory variables have already been collected at the time the investigator initiates the study. The investigator then proceeds to collect information on the outcomes of interest and retrieves the previously collected explanatory data to discover possible causal relationships. Cross-sectional studies, on the other hand, measure cause and effect variables during the same period of data collection.

Longitudinal studies are expensive, time consuming, and suffer from the effects of sample attrition over time (Greenland, 1977). Yet, in child psychiatry they represent a more powerful design in permitting one to analyze behavior as a developmental phenomenon. Numerous investigators have proposed the integration of elements of both the longitudinal and cross-sectional designs into what has been called the convergent longitudinal design (Bell, 1953), or the sequential cohort design (Schaie, 1965). An illustration of this design is shown in fig. 3 in which five age cohorts are followed over a 5-year interval. One important feature of the design is that it permits covering a longer developmental period than would be possible in the cross-sectional study. Another is that overlap of cohorts yields a larger sample size than would be obtained in a simple longitudinal design for each developmental age. Applications of this design have been few in child development research (Nesselroade and Baltes, 1974), but it is certain to be used more extensively in the future.

Ethical and Legal Considerations

Considerable efforts have been made over the past ten years in the United States to provide programmatic review of the legal and

FIGURE 3

FIVE COHORTS MEASURED AT 5 YEARLY INTERVALS

Time of Birth	Ages (in years)				
1980	4	5	6	7	8
1981	3	4	5	6	7
1982	2	3	4	5	6
1983	1	2	3	4	5
1984	-	1	2	3	4
Time of Measurement	1984	1985	1986	1987	1988

ethical issues in research involving human populations. The consequences of this development have become so far reaching that it is impossible to consider research objectives and methods without simultaneously considering their legal and ethical implications (Berger and Stallones, 1977). Intrainstitutional review committees have been established to share the burden of responsibility with investigators to protect human subjects.

At least three issues are at stake: (1) informed consent, (2) the maintenance of confidentiality, and (3) the minimization of risks. Special precautions are required in work with children because of the dual responsibility of protecting children as subjects and parents as informants.

Informed consent involves conveying the purpose of an investigation and the procedures involved in language which ensures that the parent genuinely comprehends what is at stake in the research venture. Much more is involved in the maintenance of confidentiality than removing the names of subjects or other identifying information from records or protocols before publishing the results of a study. Particularly in situations in which sensitive data about children or families are collected and stored over long intervals of time (e.g., samples of children considered at "high risk" for schizophrenia), control over access to data files must be guaranteed. In some cases the investigator will face the need to break confidentiality. For example, most states in the United States now stipulate that even suspected cases of child abuse must be reported to a designated authority (usually the state's welfare department).

Institutional review committees are required to analyze the risks and benefits of participating in a research study with the expectation that benefits will exceed risks. In psychiatric research the risks involve mental discomfort, embarrassment, and the possibility of falsely labeling a child as impaired. The benefits of participation, particularly in epidemiologic research, are ones that involve not only the individual participant (e.g., that a previously unidentified health problem becomes recognized) but also the community (e.g., by improving services).

At present, these and other legal and ethical issues involving research on human subjects are to a large extent still unresolved, resulting in a lack of uniformity between review committees and their expectations of individual research endeavors. There is a need for an open forum between investigators, review committees, and the public if a constructive resolution is to be reached which protects human subjects, but not at the expense of making important research objectives impossible. This development requires investigators to think through the ethical and legal issues likely to impact upon their work at the very beginning of research planning. When added to problems of securing research funds and recruiting samples, this additional responsibility increases the time needed to launch an epidemiologic project by several months to a year or more.

Limitations of Epidemiologic Methods

No discussion of methods is complete until the limitations and drawbacks of the sampling procedures and methods are understood and worked through. Indeed, this is one of the chief sources of labor in epidemiology. Since field surveys, particularly longitudinal ones, are expensive pursuits, it is advisable to work through improving one's methodology in clinical or laboratory settings as much as possible before embarking on large-scale field studies. Throughout this chapter, reference has been made to the variety of limitations confronting behavioral sciences in general, and epidemiology in particular. They will be briefly summarized here, but it should be emphasized that the value of this exercise is primarily bent on encouraging individual investigators to pursue such questions as a regular part of the planning and quality control of their own studies. The following are three of the chief limitations facing the epidemiologic scientist in child psychiatry:

1. A weak criterion for judging the presence and severity of psychiatric disorders which results in poor sensitivity and specificity of methods for measuring psychiatric disorder in population groups (La Pouse, 1967).
2. The multiple factorial etiology of psychiatric disorder which poses problems in research design because of the large number

of partially controlled or uncontrolled factors (Birtchnell, 1974).

3. Observer bias, beginning with theoretical biases in the underlying assumptions of a particular research design and culminating in the various forms of teacher, parent, and interviewer bias in reporting and interpreting children's behavior.

These limitations have been discussed in a variety of ways. First, the major portion of the effort in this chapter has been devoted in one way or another to issues regarding accuracy and precision, or validity and reliability of methods, of measuring behavior. The point was made that accuracy in measuring psychiatric disorder or risk factors of psychiatric disorders should be dealt with just as seriously as questions of reliability. Of the two problems in measurement, the problem of accuracy will result in the severest headache for researchers.

Secondly, of the various forms of variation encountered in measurement, systematic variation imposes the chief limitations to investigators, and if unchecked, this may result in frank drawbacks to successful research work. Finally, the analytic strategies involved in multiple factorial research designs require extensive efforts at data reduction and exploratory data analysis before embarking on the use of confirmatory statistical techniques (Tukey, 1977; Mostellar and Tukey, 1977).

New Methodological Advances

The epidemiologist shares with the clinician an ultimate concern toward understanding the meaning of emotional suffering in the child. This represents a fundamental concern for all research in child psychiatry. The epidemiologist is able to add a population perspective to etiology, natural history, duration, and distribution of behavioral problems in children. Since epidemiologic approaches in child psychiatry research are in an early stage of development with much work remaining, it is useful to forecast what methodological trends are most likely to result in new directions of research and in important findings.

An important methodological strategy is the convergence of techniques used in the definition of psychiatric disorders in children within single studies. The convergence of interview methodology, observational techniques, and physiological measurements is a largely unexplored area. While much of this exploration should take place in clinical and laboratory settings, field surveys offer the important opportunity to develop norms for new observational and physiological measurements. For example, Venables (1975) has extended the use of electrodermal skin response methodology to a prospective longitudinal field study of children. In another epidemiological study of vulnerable women with infants and young children, ethological concepts were used in developing observational measures of mother-child interaction (Wolkind, 1977). A variety of interview techniques have been developed for measuring stressful life events (Brown, 1974; Dohrenwend, 1978), and social support networks (Cassel, 1976; Dean and Lin, 1977), but little of this methodology has been translated into techniques for children. Coddington (1972) has standardized the Holmes and Rahe (1967) technique for measuring the impact of life events in adults into a methodology for children, but the technique has not been employed in an epidemiologic study, nor has it been used very extensively in a clinical setting (Heisel et al., 1973).

Recent findings suggest that very simple measures of social support can powerfully predict levels of mortality and morbidity in adults (Berkman and Syme, 1979). Translating such methodologies for use in children requires that parent-report or parent-perceptual items are incorporated, since, especially for young children, it can be assumed that life events and social support measures are to a large extent dependent upon the primary caregivers' mediation of these phenomena as part of the home environment.

A second important methodological advance is likely to take place along the lines charted recently by Bronfenbrenner (1977), discussing the concept of ecological validity. This recharting of methodologies in relationship to natural environments is certainly relevant to a fundamental improvement in the validity of methods as it attempts to insure that investigators experience similar phenomena as experienced by children, parents, and teachers. New techniques for determining validity will emerge from this new conceptual development.

Future Directions of Child Psychiatric Epidemiology

What remains is a discussion of the future directions of epidemiologic methodology for a preventive child psychiatry. Future applications of epidemiology will have somewhat different contributions to make in technologically developing countries as opposed to technologically developed countries. In emerging nations the trends of urbanization, modernization, migration, emigration, and a relatively recent emphasis on universal public education are stress factors which are qualitatively different from those in developed countries. Moreover, the interaction between social factors such as stress and biological factors such as poor nutrition and infectious disease processes increase the incidence of psychiatric disorder (Minde, 1976). The fact that the population base of children in developing countries is generally much larger proportionally than in developed countries also suggests that the burden of emotional and learning problems may be more substantial. Perhaps the developing countries can profit from the experience of the developed countries in the application of population-based techniques for administrative, scientific, and clinical studies to protect the status of children exposed to the effects of rapid modernization (Teitelbaum, 1975; Knodel, 1977). To a large extent these nations have been forced to limit their concern rather exclusively to the physical care of infants and children. Research activity and clinical services have justifiably been concentrated on problems such as the prevention of malnutrition, and on prenatal and perinatal care. In child development research in these countries an important emphasis has been placed on the recovery from the effects of damage to the brain, stemming primarily from biological insults (Cravioto and De Licardie, 1972; Birch and Gussow, 1970). Yet, it is essential, especially at a time when the infant mortality rate is decreasing in these emerging nations, to broaden health services to include aspects of the social and family environment of children. Strategies are needed to examine the extent to which social factors interact with each other and with biological factors as determinants of psychiatric morbidity.

In developed countries the application of epidemiology will be to increase knowledge on the prediction of psychiatric impairment in children at different ages, and for epidemiologic knowledge to become more solidly incorporated into clinical practice and public policy. A potential application derived from epidemiologic methodology is related to decision-making strategies (Schwartz et al., 1973; Tversky and Kahneman, 1974; Elstein, 1976). There is a long history of debate in psychology on whether clinical or statistical approaches to diagnosis are superior (Meehl, 1960; Sawyer, 1966). New directions are needed in ways of comparing and integrating these different approaches to diagnosis and decision making as in adult psychiatry, where computer based simulation of clinical judgment has been developed (Wing et al., 1974). This approach complements many of the multivariate statistical approaches to diagnosis and classification (Garside and Roth, 1978). While there are certain limitations on how far these techniques may be developed, given our current knowledge, they are exciting trends in the development of new strategies in diagnoses.

Another contribution of epidemiology regards the health screening of entire populations of children as directed by public laws in the United States (Moore, 1977). Hersh (1978) has compared the policy in Sweden with that of the United States and found the States' policy quite inferior to Sweden's, particularly in regard to the extent to which mental health evaluation techniques are incorporated. Methods derived from epidemiologic studies provide valid techniques for screening behavioral problems in children, techniques which are both time and cost efficient. Certainly, such methods should be an attractive addition to pediatric services.

It is also likely that new kinds of childhood disorders will become the focus of epidemiologic pursuits. Learning disorders in children have become the focus of intense research and clinical activity in the past ten years (Benton and Pearl, 1978); yet, important questions on causation remain. Epidemiologic approaches will have an important role to play in unraveling complex causal theories regarding this class of disorders. It appears that neurological factors play a role as distal variables and social factors assume importance as proximal variables in the causation of learning disorders. The same may be true in some forms of juvenile delinquency, although the matter is far from settled (Earls, 1978). Important new developments in the study of family resemblance of psychiatric disorders (Morten and Chung, 1978), and in the clustering of health problems in families (Newcombe, 1966; Downes and Simon, 1953) and in larger social groups (Cooper and Gath, 1977) invite contributions from epidemiologic child psychiatry. As well, new types of vulnerabilities will be recognized which contribute to an understanding of the genesis of psychiatric problems in children, such as the recently described fetal alcohol syndrome (Streissguth, 1978).

Finally, epidemiologic approaches will make important contributions to revising old theories and generating new ones. A recent effort to negate the implications of psychoanalytic theory for normative aspects of adolescent psychosexual development have been based on empirical findings from a 5-year prospective longitudinal study (Rutter et al., 1976). Findings from this study suggest that adolescence is not usually characterized by the emotional turbulence predicted by psychoanalytic theory, but that turmoil is an exceptional state of affairs more likely to come to clinical attention.

It is clear that epidemiologic methods will continue to make scientific, clinical, and administrative contributions to child psychiatry. Perhaps the most important contribution epidemiology has yet to make is in describing the extent to which emotional problems in childhood constitute a social and financial burden on human societies. Unlike the case with physical handicaps, emotional problems often go undetected because they are so thoroughly a function of the observer's judgment and interpretation. With improved physical health status of children internationally, interest in the emotional well-being of children must certainly increase. Epidemiologic methods are well suited to reveal the preponderance of emotional suffering in children, to isolate their causes, and to demonstrate their distribution in communities. As studies based on these methods accumulate, societies should be able to discharge more effectively the function of promoting the psychological health of children as an integral part of total health.

Acknowledgments

Dr. Earls's investigation is being supported by Grants MH-28266 and MH-00165 (RSDA) of the National Institute of Mental Health and in part by Core Grant HD-06276 of the Mental Retardation Center.

This paper is dedicated to Jack Tizard (1919-1979), whose compassion and integrity gave substance to epidemiologic methods in the study of handicapped children.

References

Als, H., Tronick, E., Lester, B., & Brazelton, T.B. The Brazelton Neonatal Behavioral Assessment Scale (BNBAS). *J. Abn. Child Psychol., 5*:215–231, 1977.

American Psychiatric Association, Task Force on Nomenclature and Statistics. *Diagnostic and Statistical Manual of Mental Disorders: Third Edition.* Washington, DC: American Psychiatric Association, 1978.

Barker, A.J.P. & Rose, E. *Epidemiology in Medical Practice.* New York: Churchill Livingstone, 1976.

Bell, R.Q. Convergence: An accelerated longitudinal approach. *Child Develop., 24*:145–152, 1953.

Benton, A. & Pearl, D. *Dyslexia: An Appraisal of Current Knowledge.* New York: Oxford University Press, 1978.

Berger, P.M. & Stallones, R.A. Legal liability and epidemiologic research. *Amer. J. Epid., 106*:177–183, 1977.

Berkman, L. & Syme, S. Social networks, host resistance, and mortality: A 9-year follow-up of Alameda County residents. *Amer. J. Epid., 109*:186–204, 1979.

Birch, H.G. & Gussow, J.D. *Disadvantaged Children: Health, Nutrition and School Failure.* New York: Ernne & Stration, 1970.

Birtchnell, J. Is there a scientifically acceptable alternative to the epidemiological study of familial factors in mental illness? *Soc. Sci. & Med., 8*:335–350, 1974.

Bronfenbrenner, U. Toward an experimental ecology of human development. *Amer. Psychol., 32*:513–531, 1977.

Brown, G. Meaning, measurement, and stress of life events. In: B.S. Dohrenwend & B.P. Dohrenwend (Eds.), *Stressful Life Events: Their Nature and Effects.* New York: John Wiley, 1974, pp. 217–243.

Brown, G. & Harris, T. *Social Origins of Depression: A Study of Psychiatric Disorder in Women.* London: Tavistock, Ltd., 1978.

Burt, C. *The Young Delinquent.* London: University of London Press, 1925.

Campbell, D.T. & Fiske, D.W. Convergent and discriminant validation by the multitrait-multimethod matrix. *Psychol. Bull., 56*:81–105, 1959.

Cassel, J. The contribution of the social environment to host resistance. *Amer. J. Epid., 104(2)*:107–123, 1976.

Chazan, M. & Jackson, S. Behavior problems in the infant school. *J. Child Psychol. Psychiat., 12*:199–210, 1971.

Chazan, M. & Jackson, S. Behavior problems in the infant school: Changes over two years. *J. Child Psychol. Psychiat., 15*:33–46, 1976.

Coddington, R.D. The significance of life events as etiologic factors in the diseases of children. II: A study of a normal population. *J. Psychosom. Res., 16*:205–213, 1972.

Conners, C.K. A teacher rating scale for use in drug studies with children. *Amer. J. Psychiat., 126*:884–888, 1969.

Cooper, B. & Gath, D. Psychiatric illness, maladjustment and juvenile delinquency: an ecological study in a London borough. *Psychol. Med., 7*:465–474, 1977.

Cravioto, J. & De Licardie, E. Environmental correlates of severe clinical malnutrition and language development in survivors from kwashiorkor or maramus. In: *Nutrition, the Nervous System and Behavior.* Washington, DC: Pan American Health Organization, 1972.

Cullen, K.J. A six-year controlled trial of prevention of children's behavior disorders. *J. Pediat., 88*:662–666, 1976.

Dean, A. & Lin, N. The stress-buffering role of social support. *J. Nerv. Ment. Dis., 165*:403–417, 1977.

Dohrenwend, B.S. & Dohrenwend, B.P. Some issues in research on stressful life events. *J. Nerv. Ment. Dis., 166*:7–15, 1978.

Downes, J. & Simon, K. Characteristics of psychoneurotic patients and their families as revealed in a general morbidity study. *Psychosom. Med., 15*:464–476, 1953.

Earls, F. The social reconstruction of adolescence. *Persp. Biol. Med., 22*:65–82, 1978.

Earls, F. Epidemiology and child psychiatry: historical and conceptual development. *Compr. Psychiat., 20*:256–269, 1979.

Earls, F. The prevalence of behavior problems in three-year-old children: a cross-national replication. *Arch. Gen. Psychiat.,* 1980a, in press.

Earls, F. and Richman, N. The prevalence of behavior problems in three-year-old children of West Indian-born parents. *J. Child Psychol. Psychiat., 21*:99–106, 1980b.

Earls, F. and Richman, N. Behavior problems in pre-school children of West Indian-born parents: a re-examination of family and social factors. *J. Child Psychol. Psychiat., 21*:107–117,1980c.

Eisenberg, J.G., Gersten, J.C., Langner, T.S., McCarthy, E.D., & Fagen, O. A behavioral classification of welfare children from survey data. *Amer. J. Orthopsychiat., 46*:447–463, 1976.

Elstein, A.S. Clinical judgment: psychological research and medical practice. *Science, 194*:696–700, 1976.

Ferguson, L., Partyka, L., & Lester, B. Patterns of parent perception differentiating clinic from nonclinic children. *J. Abn. Child Psychol., 2*:169–181, 1974.

Freud, S. Analysis of a Phobia in a Five Year Old Boy. In: *Complete Psychological Works, Standard Edition, Volume 10.* London: Hogarth, 1955.

Garside, R.T. & Roth, M. Multivariate statistical methods and problems of classification in psychiatry. *Brit. J. Psychiat., 133*:53–67, 1978.

Gersten, J.C., Langner, T.S., Eisenberg, J.G., Simcha-Fagan, O. & McCarthy, E.D. Stability and change in types of behavioral disturbance of children and adolescents. *J. Abn. Child Psychol.* *4*:111–127, 1976.

Glidewell, J.C., Menshi, I.N., & Gildea, M.C. Behavior symptoms in children and degree of sickness. *Amer. J. Psychiat., 114*:47–53, 1957.

Graham, P. J. Epidemiologic perspectives on maladaptation in children: neurologic, familial, and social factors. *J. Am. Acad. Child Psych., 17*:197–208, 1978.

Graham, P. J. & Rutter, M. The reliability and validity of the psychiatric assessment of the child: II. Interview with the parent. *Brit. J. Psychiat., 114*:581–592, 1968.

Greenland, S. Response and follow-up bias in cohort studies. *Amer. J. Epid., 106*:184–187, 1977.

Heisel, J.S., Ream, S., Rartz, R., Rappaport, M. & Coddington, R.D. The significance of life events as contributing factors in the diseases of children: III. a study of pediatric patients. *J. Pediat., 83*:119–123, 1973.

Hersh, S.P. Sweden's approach to health screening for preschool children. *Amer. J. Orthopsychiat., 48*:33–39, 1978.

Holmes, T.H. & Rahe, R.N. The social readjustment rating scale. *J. Psychosom. Res., 11*:213–218, 1967.

Hughes, M., Carmichael, H., Pinkerton, G. & Tizard, B. Recording children's conversations at home and at nursery school: a technique and some methodological considerations. *J. Child Psychol. Psychiat., 20*:225–232, 1979.

Ingham, J.G. & Miller, P. The concept of prevalence applied to psychiatric disorders and symptoms. *Psychol. Med., 6*:217–225, 1976.

Kellam, S.G., Branch, J.D., Agrawal, K.C. & Ensminger, M.E. *Mental Health and Going to School: The Woodlawn Program of Assessment, Early Intervention and Evaluation.* Chicago: University of Chicago Press, 1975.

Kety, S.S., Rosenthal, D., Wender, P.H. & Schulsinger, F. The types and prevalence of mental illness in the biological and adoptive families of adopted schizophrenics. In: D. Rosenthal & S.S. Kety (Eds) *The Transmission of Schizophrenia.* Oxford: Pergamon Press, 1968, pp. 345–362.

Knodel, J. Breast-feeding and population growth. *Science, 198*:1111–1115, 1977.

Langner, T.S., Gersten, J.C., Greene, E.L., Eisenberg, J.G., Herson, J.H. & McCarthy, E. Treatment of psychological disorders among urban children. *J. Consult, Clin. Psych., 42*:170–179, 1974.

La Pouse, R. The relationship of behavior to adjustment in a representative sample of children. *Amer. J. Pub. Health, 55*:1130–1141, 1965.

La Pouse, R. Problems in studying prevalence. *Amer. J. Pub. Health, 57*:947–954, 1967.

La Pouse, R. & Monk, M. An epidemiological study of behavior characteristics in children. *Amer. J. Pub. Health, 48*:1134–1144, 1958.

La Pouse, R. & Monk, M. Fears and worries in a representative sample of children. *Amer. J. Orthopsychiat., 29*:803–818, 1959.

La Pouse, R. & Monk, M. Behavior deviations in a representative sample of children: variation by sex, age, race, social class, and family size. *Amer. J. Orthopsychiat., 34*:436–446, 1964.

Leighton, A. Research directions in psychiatric epidemiology. *Psychol. Med., 9*:235–247, 1979.

Levy, D. Beginnings of the child guidance movement. *Amer. J. Orthopsychiat., 38*:799–804, 1968.

Lewis, E.O. Report on the investigation into the incidence of mental deficiency in six areas, 1925–27. In: *Report of the Mental Deficiency Committee, Part IV.* London: H.M.S.O., 1929.

MacFarlane, J.W., Allen, L. & Hauzik, M.P. *A Developmental Study of the Behavior Problems of Normal Children between 21 Months and 14 Years.* Berkeley: University of California Press, 1954.

McMahon, B. & Pugh, T.F. *Epidemiology, Principles, and Methods.* Boston: Little, Brown, & Co., 1970.

Mechanic, D. Problems and prospects in psychiatric epidemiology. In: E. H. Hare & J. K. Wing (Eds.), *Psychiatric Epidemiology.* London: Oxford University Press, 1970, pp. 3–22.

Meehl, P.E. The cognitive activity of the clinician. *Amer. Psychol., 15*:19–27, 1960.

Minde, K. K. Child psychiatry in developing countries. *J. Child Psychol. Psychiat., 17*:79–83, 1976.

Moore, B. Implementing the developmental assessment component of the EPSDT program. *Amer. J. Orthopsychiat., 47*:701–711, 1977.

Morton, N.E. & Chung, C.S. *Genetic Epidemiology.* New York: Academic Press, 1978.

Mostellar, F. & Tukey, J.W. *Data Analysis and Regression.* Reading, MA: Addison-Wesley, 1977.

Nesselroade, J. & Baltes, P. Adolescent personality development and historical change: 1970–1972. *Monogr. Soc. Res. Child Develop., 39* (1, No. 154), 1974.

Newcombe, H.B. Familial tendencies in diseases of children. *Brit. J. Prev. Soc. Med., 20*:49–57, 1966.

Richman, N. & Graham, P. J. A behavioral screening questionnaire for use with three-year-old children: preliminary findings. *J. Child Psychol. Psychiat., 12*:5–33, 1971.

Richman, N., Stevenson, J.E. & Graham, P.J. Prevalence of behavior problems in three-year-old children: an epidemiological study in a London borough. *J. Child Psychol Psychiat., 16*:277–287, 1975.

Robins, L.N. *Deviant Children Grown-up: A Sociological and Psychiatric Study of Sociopathic Personality.* Baltimore: Williams & Wilkins, 1966.

Robins, L.N. Sturdy childhood predictors of adult antisocial behavior: replications from longitudinal studies. *Psychol. Med., 8*:611–622, 1978.

Rogan, W.J. & Gladen, B. Estimating prevalence from the results of a screening test. *Amer. J. Epid., 107*:71–76, 1978.

Rutter, M. Children's behavior questionnaire for completion by teachers: Preliminary findings. *J. Child Psychol. Psychiat., 8*:1–11, 1967.

Rutter, M. Relationships between child and adult psychiatric disorder. *Acta Psych. Scand. 48*:3–21, 1972.

Rutter, M., Cox, A., Tupling, C., Berger, M. & Yule, W. Attainment and adjustment in two geographical areas. *Brit. J. Psychiat., 126*:493–509, 1975(b).

Rutter, M. & Graham, P. The reliability and validity of the psychiatric assessment of the child: I. Interview with the child. *Brit. J. Psychiat., 114*:563–579, 1968.

Rutter, M., Graham, P., Chadwick, O. & Yule, W. Adolescent turmoil—fact or fiction? *J. Child Psychol. Psychiat., 17*:35–56, 1976.

Rutter, M., Graham, P. & Yule, W. A neuropsychiatric study in childhood. *Clinics in Develop. Med.* (Numbers 35, 36), 1970(b).

Rutter, M., Shaffer, D. & Shepherd, M. *A Multiaxial Classification of Child Psychiatric Disorders*: An Evaluation of a Proposal. Geneva: World Health Organization, 1975(a).

Rutter, M., Tizard, J. & Whitmore, K. *Education, Health and Behaviour.* London: Longmans, 1970(a).

Sameroff, A.J. (Ed.) Organization and stability of newborn behavior: A commentary on the Brazelton Neonatal Behavior Assessment Scale. *Mon. S.R.C.D.*, *43*(5–6, Serial No. 177), 1979.

Sameroff, A.J. & Chandler, M.J. Reproductive risk and the continuum of caretaking casualty. In: F.D. Horowitz, M. Hetherington, S. Scarr-Salapatek, & G. Siegel (Eds.), *Review of Child Development Research,* Chicago: University of Chicago, 1975, *4*:187–244.

Sawyer, J. Measurement and prediction: Clinical and statistical. *Psychol. Bull.*, *66*:178–200, 1966.

Schaie, F.W., A general model for the study of developmental problems. *Psychol. Bull.*, *64*:92–107, 1965.

Schwartz, W.B., Gorry, G.A., Kassner, J.P. & Essig, A. Decision analysis and clinical judgment. *Amer. J. Med.*, *55*:459–472, 1973.

Shepherd, M., Oppenheim, A.N. & Mitchell, S. Childhood behavior disorders and the child-guidance clinic: An epidemiological study. *J. Child Psychol. Psychiat.*, *7*:39–52, 1966.

Shrout, P.E. & Fleiss, J.L. Intraclass correlations: Uses in assessing rater reliability. *Psychol. Bull.*, *86*:420–428, 1979.

Streissguth, A.P. Fetal alcohol syndrome: An epidemiologic perspective. *Amer. J. Epid.*, *107*:467–478, 1978.

Teitelbaum, M.S. Relevance of demographic transition theory for developing countries. *Science, 188*:420–425, 1975.

Terris, M. The score and methods of epidemiology. *Amer. J. Pub. Health*, *52*:1371–1376, 1962.

Tukey, J.W. *Exploratory Data Analysis.* Reading, MA: Addison-Wesley, 1977.

Tversky, A. & Kahneman, D. Judgment under uncertainty: Heuristics and biases. *Science, 185*:1124–1131, 1974.

Venables, P.H. Progress in psychophysiology: Some applications in a field of abnormal psychology. In: P.H. Venables & M.J. Christie (Eds.), *Progress in Psychophysiology.* New York: John Wiley, 1975, pp. 418–437.

Wickman, E.K. *Children's Behavior and Teachers' Attitudes.* New York: Commonwealth Fund, 1928.

Wing, J.K., Cooper, J.E., & Sartorius, N. *The Measurement and Classification of Psychiatric Symptoms.* London: Cambridge University Press, 1974.

Wing, J.K., Mann, S.A., Leff, J.P. & Nixon, J.M. The concept of a "case" in psychiatric population surveys. *Psychol. Med.*, *8*:203–217, 1978.

Wolkind, S., Hall, F. & Pawlby, S. Individual differences in mothering behavior: A combined epidemiological and observational approach. In: P. Graham (Ed.), *Epidemiologic Approaches in Child Psychiatry.* London: Academic Press, pp. 107–123, 1977.

Wright, S. The application of path analysis to etiology. In: N.E. Morton & C.S. Chung (Eds.), *Genetic Epidemiology.* New York: Academic Press, pp. 13–51, 1978.

Zimmerman-Tansella, C., Mingheth, S., Tacconi, A. & Tansella, M. The children's behavior questionnaire for completion by teachers in an Italian sample: Preliminary results. *J. Child Psychol. Psychiat.*, *19*:167–173, 1978.

Longitudinal Methods in the Study of Normal and Pathological Development

LEE N. ROBINS, PH.D.

What is a Longitudinal Study?

A longitudinal study differs from other studies in only one respect: it involves measures taken at two or more points in time. The things measured may be of the same or different kinds. That is, we may repeat a measurement from Time 1 and Time 2 in an attempt, for instance, to see whether IQs change over time, or we may look at different kinds of behaviors in the same people.

Design for this Chapter

The chapter examines the follow-up study as a method for learning about the normal and abnormal development of children. The chapter will cover the purposes for which longitudinal studies of children have been used, various follow-up study designs and their advantages and hazards, methods for the selection of samples, the use of control subjects, what data about the Time 1 period need to be gathered, the length of the follow-up interval, measures appropriate for describing Time 2 (outcome), and problems of interpretation and presentation of results. These topics will be illustrated by examples from some important follow-up studies. To illustrate the power of follow-up studies of children, the chapter will conclude with findings from some of these studies, particularly those findings that have been replicated in studies in different kinds of samples and different eras. Thus the chapter will make sense at two levels: as a technical guide to considerations that one should keep in mind when planning a follow-up study, and as a substantive report that will illustrate some of the things that follow-up studies have done and some of the common-sense knowledge they have shown to be myths.

Questions Attacked by Follow-Up Studies

One area to which follow-up studies of children have made a major contribution is in the description of the development of children or young people over time. Some of these studies have begun in early infancy or even before birth, by enlisting the cooperation of pregnant women. An example of the last is the Fels Institute Project (Study E), which began observing women from the time of identified pregnancy and then followed the children into adulthood. Longitudinal studies of normal development are usually distinguished by their frequent periods of observation. Examples of these are the Thomas and Chess study (Study V), which began looking at infants immediately after birth and followed them at intervals into their teens. The earliest classic study of this type was the Berkeley Growth Study (Study A), which began with very young children and followed them into their thirties. Although the tactical problems are enormous, a few such studies have included very large samples: 55,000 in the USA collaborative perinatal study (Niswander and Gordon, 1972), and 16,000 in the British National Child Development Study (Study P). While prospective studies of normal populations from infancy on have included some psychological components, they are not exclusively interested in psychiatric problems and psychological development. In addition to such interests, they have been concerned with physical and intellectual development, educational achievement, and predictors of occupational performance.

Other follow-up studies have sought prognosticators of pathology, defined as psychiatric symptoms, poor functioning in school, or delinquency. Some studies were intended to illuminate the effects of particular agents thought to be causative agents such as genetic loading for psychiatric disorder, pathological family environment, mother's absence, early toilet training, or adoption. These studies have been cast in a quasi-experimental model to contrast children exposed and not exposed to the presumed cause.

Another important use of follow-up studies has been a nosological one. Psychiatry, lacking laboratory tests for the presence or absence of illness, has relied on follow-up studies to provide validity parameters for diagnosis. If children given a particular diagnosis always either continue to show that same diagnosis at a later age or recover from it, this constitutes evidence for the existence of that diagnosis as a discrete syndrome. If, on the other hand, children so diagnosed typically develop some other well-known diagnostic entity later on, this constitutes evidence that the diagnosis in childhood was not discrete but only the more familiar adult disorder in an early, undeveloped stage. Similarly, if the offspring of adults with a given diagnosis turn out to have a higher rate than expected of that same diagnosis, and a rate no higher than expected of any other diagnosis, this constitutes evidence for the reality of the adult diagnosis, since it must be capable of being passed on either genetically, by modelling, or by subjecting the offspring to the same environment that produced the disorder in the parent's case. Follow-up studies thus can provide important clues to the integrity of a diagnostic entity, as opposed to its being a transient reactive state or simply a variant of another diagnosis. Stability of findings longitudinally has also been used to argue the importance of personality traits and to argue that IQ scores are indicators of inborn capacity. (Scientists are, of course, still challenging the IQ test's validity as such an indicator. Stability alone does not *prove* its validity, but instability would have been sufficient to disprove it.)

Longitudinal studies are also useful for the simple measurement of the prevalence of psychiatric disorders, personality traits, or intelligence. While this is a cross-sectional question essentially, longitudinal studies have advantages, as we will discuss later, in guaranteeing a representative sample of the population. They can also provide rates of expected incidence of new problems in order to predict future needs, with no causal hypotheses in mind. They may be hypothesis generating, looking through a vast array of variables for predictors of specific outcomes. They may be looking at traumatic events to see to which of a host of outcomes they might contribute. They may be designed to test a very specific hypothesis generated by a cross-sectional study or a longitudinal study in a different population. Finally, they may be experiments in the truest sense when, for instance, they assess the effectiveness of treatment by comparing children randomly assigned to control or treated cohorts. In such cases they differ from the classic laboratory experiment only in the relatively long elapsed time between the beginning and the end of the study and in the greater difficulties of keeping all nonexperimental variables under control.

Typical Designs of Follow-Up Studies

Considering the broad range of purposes that follow-up studies of children can serve, it is not surprising that they also encompass a variety of study designs, some more appropriate for one, some for another purpose. Within the diversity of possible follow-up designs there are three main types: the real-time prospective study, the follow-back study, and the "catch-up" prospective study.

The "Real-Time" Prospective Study—The real-time prospective study selects a sample at Time 1, examines its members, and then either waits to measure again at Time 2 or interjects an experiment in treatment or prevention that is supposed to change the measures at reassessment at Time 2. The real-time prospective study is the only one that can provide researcher-designed evaluation at Time 1 or at multiple points between entry into the study and termination. It is usually the only acceptable design for therapeutic trials, not only because its baseline measures meet research criteria, but also because it allows random assignment to alternative treatments and to no treatment. When membership in the treatment or control group is not rigorously controlled by random assignment, entry into treatment is likely to be correlated with outcome variables. Children who enter treatment voluntarily are presumably sicker than those who refuse it, and among those equally in need of treatment, those who actually enter it are more likely to come from those social strata with greater faith in ameliorative efforts, usually the educated middle class.

Despite these advantages, the prospective design should be avoided whenever possible. It has other problems that often more than make up for its virtues. One difficulty with prospective follow-up studies of children is that children age slowly as compared with most other experimental animals, and indeed as slowly as the experimenter. This means that questions of long-term outcome are difficult to answer within the lifespan of a single investigator. And even were he so durable and persistent as to stick with his project until all his child subjects were adult, by the time he is ready to do his final evaluation of his now mature cohort, he finds that science has also matured. Those very careful measurements he took 30 years ago look crude in the light of the new tools available, and the very dimensions he chose to measure may no longer interest him or the rest of the scientific community. The place for the real-time prospective longitudinal study is in reasonably short-term studies, studies in which highly reliable repeated outcome measures are necessary, studies involving a true experiment in which the researcher must provide the experimental intervention as well as the before and after assessments, or where there are no available routine measurements at Time 1 from which adequate baseline figures can be prepared. If these requirements *are* realistic, there is no choice but to start a prospective study, unless one is lucky enough to find one started some time ago by another researcher who has since given up but still has the baseline data of the kind needed. Where the problem requires a prospective study of long duration, the researcher had better be sure that is what he wants to do with the rest of his career. In the U.S., there are studies still in progress that have lasted more than thirty years. Retiring researchers have passed their data on to their juniors, some of whom are now themselves reaching retirement age. Among the studies with such longevity are the Berkeley Growth Study (A), the Fels Study (E), the Cambridge–Somerville Youth Study (C), and the Terman Study of Gifted Children (U). Only one of these, the Cambridge–Somerville Youth Study, was a treatment study. It has continued long past the time needed for evaluation of treatment, but has been maintained nonetheless because of the wealth of data collected during the treatment phase.

Many studies must be prospective because the data needed at Time 1 are not routinely available. Thus Rutter's study of Isle of Wight children (T1) required a psychiatric evaluation of a total population at the initial point in time. His study shows one way of reducing the risks involved in prospective studies. Because it was the first study to apply diagnostic criteria to a complete population of children, it was a valuable cross-sectional study at Time 1. Even had he failed to carry out the follow-up component, it would have been well worth doing.

In addition to the waiting time problem mentioned above, real-time prospective studies with multiple points of evaluation involve another difficulty—the problem of maintaining the sample. When children are to be repeatedly evaluated, one must keep them and their parents pleased with their participation. This goal may seriously limit (or, which is just as serious, be believed by the investigators to limit) the range of questions that can be asked and measures that can be taken. Thus, real-time prospective studies are distinguished by their avoidance of materials that might be thought to be embarrassing or incriminating.

Prospective studies are often designed around repeated assessments at fixed intervals. Monitoring changes every few months or every year is often thought to be a technique for precisely assessing cause-effect relationships between changes in environment and their reflections in behavior. In practice, unfortunately, carrying out this design is always difficult and sometimes misleading. One can be misled because frequent repetition of measures maximizes practice effects, effects which have been shown by Baltes et al. (1972) to apply to a variety of psychological instruments. Thus true changes may be greater or less than repeated measurement indicates. Second, it is always difficult to carry out the assessments within as short a time span as necessary if the intervals between tests are to be approximately the same for all subjects. The investigator usually has to choose between incomplete recovery of his cases for a particular assessment or stretching the permissible interval during which that particular assessment occurs. This latter choice means that the interval between assessments 2 and 3, for example, may be considerably shorter than planned for children who at Time 2 were difficult to locate or to arrange an appointment for. Such distortions in the planned interval mean that children are not all the expected ages at evaluation and have not all had the same period of risk between evaluations.

Finally, as children develop, the same test forms do not remain appropriate. Since different test forms for different ages are never perfectly equivalent, one may find oneself trying to explain fluctuations on the microlevel that have no real meaning in terms of the contributions of predictors to clinically important levels of life adjustment. Knowing too much detail can indeed blind the investigator to his major results.

These difficulties often compromise the original scheme sufficiently to make repeated assessments both more expensive and less valuable than anticipated. Indeed, they may be practical only when they can be attached to routine occasions in the child's life, such as the annual school health examination.

Because repeated evaluations are expensive, prospective studies that require them have often used samples of only moderate size. When the inevitable sample losses between multiple evaluations occur, the sample becomes both too small and too unrepresentative of the initial population to draw conclusive inferences, despite the richness of detail for each case. Thus in the combined Berkeley Youth Study (A), when evaluated by Block (1971), there were only 171 cases left of 460.

There are certain longitudinal studies for which a real-time prospective design would be particularly inappropriate, even were it not so difficult and lengthy to carry out. When the goal of the study is to understand predictors of rare events or conditions, it is especially uneconomical to study prospectively the large sample necessary to get enough cases of the outcome of interest at a later date. To obtain enough cases to study a rare outcome prospectively, one generally must resort to choosing the sample from a high-risk population, a population in which the outcome is not so rare. But the price one then pays is omission of those cases with atypical backgrounds. An alternative is the follow-back design.

The "Follow-Back" Study—The follow-back design chooses as its index cases those already known to have the rare outcome. It then requires locating earlier records about each case and comparing them with records made at the same time for appropriate control cases. Differences between the two are interpreted as indicating either causes of the disorder or its early unrecognized signs. An example of this type is Watt's (Study W) study of a population of persons admitted to psychiatric hospitals for a functional disorder between the ages of 15 and 35, whose records were located in the public school records of one town. The school record of each hospitalized case was compared with the record of a control case attending the same school and similar to those later hospitalized in age, sex, and social status. The study focused on predictors of schizophrenia, a disorder estimated to occur in only 0.8% of the school population. A prospective study starting with a random sample of school children clearly would not have been practical. To get the number of schizophrenics obtained by the methods used would have required examining all 9600 students enrolled during this period, instead of the small sample actually used, and waiting many years for them to have passed through the risk period for schizophrenia. Follow-back studies have much to offer in terms of economics of time and money.

In the Watt study, both early and late information was obtained only from records, so the researcher had no contact with the patients at all—he merely linked existing records and harvested his reward inexpensively. The saving in time and effort is attractive but has its scientific costs. All follow-back studies share the disadvantage of having to rely on existing measures for Time 1 data. Watt also relied on existing records for Time 2 data. In principle, the follow-back design does not prevent the researcher from applying his own measuring devices at Time 2—in this case, precise diagnostic criteria. But this would have greatly increased costs for Watt, since he included cases no longer in the hospital. He would have had to locate and interview them at home, and would still have been faced with the problem of making a diagnosis retrospectively for those found to be in remission.

An additional drawback of the follow-back study is that it requires access to an unbiased population of those with the disorder of interest if one's study is to apply to everyone with the disorder. There are few psychiatric problems other than schizophrenia and severe mental retardation for which a reasonably representative sample is likely to be available in any register or other set of records. If this method were applied to disorders where care is optional, one might very well be identifying in childhood records predictors of seeking care rather than predictors of the disorder itself. There would be no way to disentangle the two.

Finally, the follow-back study usually provides no estimate of how many cases have been missed among those whose records *should* have been available at Time 1. Watt, for instance, defined his sample as persons with records in both the psychiatric register and the schools. He has no way of knowing whether he failed to locate some patients who actually attended those schools, since hospital records of older persons do not usually specify their place of residence some years before. This *may* be of no practical importance, but if more disturbed young people were in school so briefly that their records were incomplete and unavailable, he may be underestimating early differences between patients and controls.

"Catch-Up" Prospective Studies—A third study design, which combines the features of the prospective and follow-back studies, is what we might call a "catch-up" prospective study. In this design, as in the real-time prospective study, the sample is identified as of Time 1, but like the follow-back study, Time 1 data come from existing records. The researcher chooses his sample from records that have already "aged" before the research begins, so that he can begin the follow-up immediately. This design eliminates the waiting period without sacrificing the opportunity to choose an unbiased sample of the population of interest. However, the researcher must sacrifice the opportunity to administer initial and interval evaluations himself.

This method has been used for a variety of studies. Adoption studies (e.g., Study D) and other studies of offspring of psychiatric patients have used the "catch-up" design because a real-time prospective study would have required a whole generation's waiting time before the offspring would have passed through the age of risk for the parents' disorder. In many studies, old records of adoptions and of parents' hospitalizations or incarcerations provided the population from which the sample was selected. Then records concerning the offspring were sought, and in some cases the adoptive parents and mature offspring located and interviewed.

When one can be satisfied with the quality of records for both time periods, the catch-up prospective study is as economical as the follow-back method. It differs from the follow-back procedure only in selecting the sample on the basis of Time 1 rather than Time 2 records. Using record information at both time periods is satisfactory when the Time 1 roster is a complete population (e.g., all births or all adoptions), so that one can be sure to have chosen a representative sample, and when the Time 2 records are complete and accurate. An example is the study of the later school achievement of legally adopted children (Seglow et al., Study P), since by definition all legal adoptions must have been recorded by the courts and because school achievement is itself defined by what appears in school records.

Often, however, records are not satisfactory sources of outcome data when the outcome variables are not routinely measured for the whole population—for instance, psychological or physiological test scores—or when the outcome is a general one such as social adjustment or psychiatric status. Available records identify only the extreme cases of social adjustment and psychiatric status. At the failure end, one finds records of detected criminals and those psychiatrically disturbed enough to come to a psychiatrist's attention. At the success end, one finds the famous among biographical listings of notables. Appearance in records even for the extreme cases may be biased by irrelevant social factors, such as the size of the police force in the local town. Further, the data found in existing records may be too inaccurate to meet research criteria, as psychiatric diagnoses in hospital records often are. When any of these conditions exists, the researcher's follow-up must include personal contact to allow administering tests or interviews. Locating cases and making individual measurements greatly increase costs, but even with this expense, catch-up prospective studies are still much less expensive than are real-time prospective studies.

One of the ways in which the catch-up study can be useful is in providing the proper sampling frame for studies in which change over time is not an issue, but the choice of an unbiased sample is. In studying the prevalence of deviant behavior, it is common to do area sampling, based on household enumerations. Yet one of the most striking findings about troubled people is that they are much less likely to be found in households than is the rest of the population. They have higher death rates, higher rates of incarceration and hospitalization, more time out of the house even when they are officially in residence, and some have no fixed address. Samples chosen from rosters of births and early school records, rosters created before the deviant behavior began, provide a truly representative sample, which when followed, yields more accurate estimates of the number of psychiatrically ill or deviant in a population than do area samples. The more deviant are still less likely to be found at home, but at least the researcher knows that they exist and must be searched for.

In addition to providing a sample which is not biased against deviant behavior and illness, sample selection from an early general population roster allows choosing samples homogenous or stratified along those dimensions for which information is recorded in the roster. Thus one can choose samples with special age and sex distributions from birth or school rosters to test particular hypotheses.

In the United States and other countries lacking national registers, the catch-up prospective design is more feasible for studies of general samples of children than of adults, since virtually all children must register at school before age seven, but never again do *all* enter any set of records. For both children and adults, various agency records can also serve if the sample desired is a special-purpose one, rather than a general sample of the population.

Rosters can provide not only a sampling frame, but also information about the subjects selected up to the age at which they enter the sample. Whichever sample design is chosen, unless Time 1 is the moment of birth, some retrospective data for the period preceding Time 1 is usually collected. When Time 1 records are not sufficiently complete, this is done by retrospective interviewing either at Time 1 for real-time prospective studies, or at Time 2 for catch-up studies. Retrospective interviewing about the period prior to Time 1 not only enriches the evaluation of the subjects at Time 1, but can also provide hypotheses to test during follow-up. As an example, in a prospective study of drug use among students (Study K), Kandel found at Time 1 that best friends of users also tended to be users. She then predicted that at follow-up those who were not yet users at Time 1 but whose friends were already using, would become users before follow-up.

Selecting the Index Sample

We have described three alternatives in follow-up study design, and pointed out that the choice among them depends on the particular problem the study is trying to answer. Of course, the same criterion determines the type of population the study sample should be chosen to represent. Samples of children who have been included in longitudinal studies have represented populations of the intellectually gifted (Study U); normal children (Studies A, E, H, J, K, M, P, Q, T1, V, X, Y, and Z); children not known to have any pathology at time of selection but thought to have a high future risk of deviance or psychiatric problems because of their race, social class, and sex (the Head Start children in Study O, the black school boys in Study R2, the inner city children in Study T1), because of their parents' problems (the offspring of criminals in Study D1, offspring of schizophrenic mothers in Study N, the children of impoverished, low-IQ mothers in Study 1), or because of their unusual family structure (the adopted children in Studies F and P); and deviant children (the Child Guidance Clinic samples in Studies R1 and S, the reformatory sample in Study G, the boys nominated by teachers as likely to get into trouble in Study C, the hyperactive boys in Study B, the autistic children in Study T2).

When the sample is of gifted or deviant children, the motivation is obvious—to find out how these unusual children turn out later on. When the population is an unselected one, the interest has rather been in describing normal development or in getting accurate incidence figures for common types of problems such as delinquency. Only when general samples are extremely large can they also be used to estimate the incidence of rare problems, like severe mental retardation or cerebral palsy. High-risk samples allow the researcher to explore a variety of possible causes of relatively rare outcomes. General samples are not ordinarily useful for this purpose because if small they would yield too few cases to test causal hypotheses and if very large, the individual cases could not be studied intensively enough to compare the impact of more than a few factors.

Homogeneity vs. Heterogeneity—In addition to choosing the type of sample—advantaged, normal, disadvantaged, or deviant—the researcher must decide how much heterogeneity he will allow in demographic variables. *Unplanned* heterogeneity may leave the researcher with too few cases of the types in which he is especially interested to get stable estimates.

Definition of the population to be studied is the major way of limiting the heterogeneity of the follow-up sample. The population can be limited to one sex, one race, a narrow age range, or residence in a particular location. Once the population is described, the researcher must accept whatever natural heterogeneity occurs within that population. Restricting the age range simplifies many problems of follow-ups of children. Children grow so rapidly that a sample spanning even a few years may not all be testable in the same manner. Some may be too young to be interviewed themselves, and so must be evaluated through interviews with parents, while others are old enough for interviews. Those personally interviewable will not find the same questions appropriate if they vary in age, and the same findings will have different significance for children of different ages—as bed wetting and night fears are normal in young children but symptoms in older children. Psychological tests are often designed for children of specific ages, with alternate forms for various ages that may not be truly equivalent.

Despite the great convenience of limiting follow-ups to narrow age spans, there are times when this is neither practical nor desirable. When the sample is to be selected from a small population, the requirement of homogeneity in age or other characteristics may yield too small a sample. But even if the need for sufficient cases did not force one to extend the age range, there are very real advantages of including more than one age cohort in the follow-up, as Baltes has shown (1968). Multiple cohorts allow the testing of findings from one cohort in another. Replication between cohorts is the best evidence of a solid finding. Cohorts born in different years also provide an opportunity to judge whether historical changes are affecting the variables of interest. If historical changes are occurring, prevalence rates at the same ages should differ among age cohorts, even though the same correlates of those rates may be found. To demonstrate that such changes over time are not due to sampling error, one needs more than two cohorts, to show linear changes or to show that peaking of prevalence occurs in certain *years* rather than at certain *ages*. As an example of an issue that needs to be addressed by multiple cohorts, there is the question of whether or not there has been a heroin epidemic in the United States. If there has been, one expects that most heroin use would have begun in the same calendar year, among young people within a relatively broad range of age at risk. With a single age cohort, it would not be possible to distinguish the effect of age at risk of beginning heroin use from the effect of the epidemic. O'Donnell et al. (1976), by following registrants with Selective Service Boards over an eight-year interval, were able to separate out *age* of initiation from *year* of initiation. It should be noted, however, that when multiple age cohorts are used, it is necessary that the ages at which outcomes are evaluated *must overlap* among the cohorts, because it is only during the overlapping years of age that the cohorts can be compared. An interesting example of this design is the Fels Study (E), in which small successive cohorts of children were admitted at birth each year. This study now makes possible discovering secular changes in developmental timing.

Simple Random vs. Stratified Samples—If one knows ahead of time what the important variables are likely to be, there are great advantages in oversampling from those portions of the population that are relatively rare but have important characteristics. In studying the effect of school problems, for instance, if one believes outcomes may differ by sex, it may be necessary to oversample those girls with problems since school problems are less common in girls than boys. For similar reasons, Robins (Study R2) and Douglas (Study Q) oversampled school children of upper and middle class backgrounds, because a sample in which their appearance was proportional to their appearance in the general population would have produced too few cases for separate analysis. So long as one knows the sampling fraction for each stratum selected, oversampling those of special interest does not prevent estimates for the total population. Each stratum can simply be weighted appropriately.

Available Sources for Identifying Index Cases

Among the sources that have served researchers in choosing index cases with which to conduct longitudinal studies of children are birth records (Studies A, B, and Q), hospital records (Studies L, N, and W), military records (Study S), school records (Studies R2, U, and Y), records of social welfare and adoption agencies (Studies D, M, and P), child guidance clinic records (Study R1), police records (Study D1), institutions of the criminal justice system (Study G), surveys of parents and teachers (Studies I, M, and T1), national health registers of psychiatric care and adoption (Study D), and populations in school classrooms (Studies H, K, and Z).

Whether or not a source of index subjects is the appropriate one depends on the degree to which it provides an unbiased sample of the population to which one wishes to extrapolate results, its ability to provide samples appropriate to testing the particular hypotheses of the study, and its accuracy in providing the identifiers necessary to locate the subject in other records or for personal interview.

Records of agencies dealing with human problems—e.g., mental institutions, child guidance clinics, courts, welfare agencies—typically see the more extreme cases along the spectrum of human troubles, while milder cases often go without official notice. Thus, reformatory children chosen by the Gluecks' (Study G) were more severely deviant than are most delinquents known to the courts, and delinquents known to the courts are in turn more serious offenders than the typical child known to the police, who is himself more seriously deviant than is the typical child who commits some illegal act. Similarly, welfare cases do not represent all children reared in poverty. Thus, while agency records are excellent sources of cases when the goal of the study is to find outcomes or predictors of *severe* problems, using them alone limits the ability to generalize to all levels of difficulty.

We noted earlier that area samples are unsatisfactory for the identification of unbiased samples of adults because the more seriously disturbed cases will be missed. While this makes them a poor source of cases for follow-back studies which start with adults, they are satisfactory for identifying young children. The dependence of young children on their parents means that virtually all of them are members of households. Those missing include the small number who are severely retarded, psychotic, or seriously physically ill, and those institutionalized because of their parents' problems or deaths. For follow-up studies of older children and adolescents, the problems outlined for adults begin to apply. Increasingly with age, those missed will be the more deviant.

Thus for real-time prospective studies of general populations of young children, birth records, school records, teacher nominations, and area samples are all acceptable sources. For catch-up prospective studies, early school or birth records are the best sources for general samples or children with school problems, and rosters covering the total population at risk, such as national adoption records, are the best source for studies of high-risk children. Secondary school records are a more biased source of general populations than are elementary school records, since some children will have dropped out of school before reaching high school. Appropriate area samples do not exist for catch-up studies, because there are no records preserved of past neighborhood memberships from which to sample.

Follow-back strategies, attractive as they are for identifying sufficient cases of rare problems, are based on cases selected from special agency records, and thus exclude the milder cases. One way to broaden the range of severity if the index case is to be interviewed is to ask him to identify relatives who had similar pathology. Since psychiatric disorders run in families, there are likely to be such relatives available, many of whom will be milder cases who have not been entered into any treatment agency's records. They can then be interviewed to verify the diagnosis and followed backward into childhood records and compared with a control case just as the original sample is followed.

How and When to Choose Control Cases

A study of a random sample of a total population such as all the children in a schoolroom or all the children on the Isle of Wight (Study T1) produces its own index and control groups: the children who at follow-up are found to have problems form an index group which can be contrasted with children who are found to be well-adjusted, the control group. Earlier measures can then be scanned for variables that differentiate between them. In the Jessors' (Study J) annual follow-up of school children over a four-year school period, control groups to compare with children who began various deviant behaviors—sex, drinking, smoking marijuana—in the last year were drawn from those who had also entered that year with no previous experience with the activity but who did *not* begin it.

When the sample is not representative of a general population, but only of one section of it—whether a section expected to have more or less difficulty then the general population—the question arises as to whether a control group is necessary. If the goal is to evaluate whether the outcomes of that section of the population are actually worse or better than the general population's and how much worse or better, we usually need one. The exception is when the distribution of the outcome measure in the general population is already known. At present, national norms are widely available for a few psychological tests and for some educational achievement tests, but norms for most other kinds of measures—coming to treatment, symptom levels, trouble with the police—are not available.

Even when tests for which national norms are available are to be used as outcome measures, control subjects may be necessary, since the index cases are likely to differ from the general population along dimensions correlated with test results. For instance, adoptees live largely in middle-class families (Study P), and in the United States include few children from ethnic minority groups. Since class and ethnic group are correlated with IQ and school achievement, failure to select a comparison group from similar environments would underestimate the disability associated with adoption.

If our intention is to show that certain subgroups of index cases differ from others rather than to compare outcomes (or origins in a follow-back study) of index cases with general population rates, it may not be necessary to have a normal control group. Rutter and Lockyer (Study T2), for instance, used a patient control group in their follow-up of autistic children. The latter's handicap was so gross that there was no need to prove that their outcomes were worse than those of normal children. Given that autistic children become severely impaired adolescents and adults, Rutter looked *within* the autistic sample for variables that distinguished those with the worst outcomes from those with less bad outcomes, creating an internal comparison group based on outcomes.

In treatment studies, it is customary to provide an untreated control group for contrast. Both groups are children with initial problems, half randomly assigned to treatment, the other half to no treatment. Baseline measures of severity of disorder are taken in both groups. The better studies of this type provide some sham treatment for the controls to rule out the simple effects of attention and enthusiasm. When the index group has completed its treatment, the two groups are readministered the same test. If the index group shows more change in a positive direction than the control group, the treatment is judged effective.

The difficulty with such treatment studies, as commonly carried out, is that they pay little attention to the *quantity* of improvement that can be attributed to the treatment, and they do not provide a second important control group—normals. Treatments always have costs. Unless the benefits can be shown to be *substantial,* the treatment may not be worth the trouble even if it has been shown statistically to lead to more improvement than does no treatment. The value of a normal group is to make it possible to quantify how close to normal the treated child has become. This quantification is worthwhile even when there is no expectation that treatment will make a disturbed child entirely normal, since it allows comparison of one treatment with another.

What constitutes a normal control group is not always self-evident. Mednick et al. (1971) studied birth complications as related to schizophrenia by assessing the hospital records of schizophrenics' children, using other births at the same hospital as a control group. They found no excess complications, except for lower birth weight. Only later did they (Mednick et al., 1973) discover that that hospital specialized in births to two kinds of mothers: unwed mothers, and those referred because their doctors expected the births to be complicated. Since 62% of the schizophrenics' children were illegitimate, it was not surprising that they had no excess birth complications as compared with controls!

The type of error Mednick et al. encountered often occurs in studies where the control group is the remainder of a treatment population—and it is an error that is almost never recognized. What appears to be a distinguishing problem or asset of the index cases may simply be an indication of the abnormal *absence* of that problem or asset in the rest of the treatment population. The important thing to remember is that there has to be *some* pathology to account for the control group's being treated. The mere fact that the rest of the treated population is more heterogeneous than the index cases is no guarantee that it is like the general population in the relevant dimension.

When the decision is made to choose a control group from the general population, there are still a number of options as to its nature. The major alternatives are a simple random sample of the population, a random sample from which all affected cases have been removed, a sample matched to the index cases on various demographic variables, or siblings. Which of these alternatives to select depends on which is least likely to create spurious findings. The correctness of the results will depend on whether differences discovered between the index cases and controls can safely be interpreted as explained by the variables that have been chosen for study variables such as symptoms, treatment experience, or family characteristics. If these variables happen to be correlated with uncontrolled variables such as sex, age, or socioeconomic group, spurious findings may occur. That is, differences between index and control cases that we attribute to the variables we *have* identified may actually be attributable to these unidentified correlates. To reduce the risk of spurious conclusions, the researcher can either choose control subjects who match the index cases on possible confounding variables or he can select a random control group and impose statistical controls later. (Even when matched cases are chosen, possible confounding correlates may turn up later which require statistical control.)

In longitudinal studies of index children undergoing a change in environment, as do adoptees, children who enter treatment or correctional institutions, and children who suffer the loss of a parent, it is valuable to have two control groups—one reflecting the earlier and one the later environment. However, both need to be appropriately matched with the index group—either by selection or by statistical control. Crellin et al. (Study P) compared adopted illegitimate children's early school success with the achievement of both nonadopted illegitimate children and legitimate children living with their natural parents. The adoptees did better than the non-adopted illegitimate controls and worse than the legitimate controls. However, the nonadopted controls were raised in much poorer families and the legitimate controls in somewhat poorer families than the adoptees. When statistical controls for social status of rearing are applied, the advantage of the adopted over the un-adopted illegitimate controls disappears in the only class level in which there are reasonably large samples of both groups (Class III), and the disadvantage of adoptees as compared with legitimate controls disappears in the white-collar families, suggesting either that white-collar families have skills and resources to overcome the handicap of adoption or that they are given infants with lower initial handicap, or both.

In follow-up studies of children treated for psychiatric problems, because it is recognized that patient status itself may affect outcome, the appropriate control group is often thought to be child patients without known psychological problems. The difficulty is that we are learning that there are intimate associations between the physical and emotional health of children. A favorite patient control group is children with fractures, since they are not "sick." However, more aggressive and daring children as well as less well-coordinated children have more injuries, and thus children with injuries are not a random sample of normal children who just "accidentally" happen to be in the hospital.

Before deciding to use matched rather than randomly chosen controls, it is important to remember that any variable used in the matching process is then lost to the analysis. The Glueck research (Study G), which found a strong association between family structure and delinquency, was severely criticized for having matched controls to delinquents on ethnic background and social status on the one hand, and on the other for *failing* to match on school enrollment. (Since the control subjects were chosen from schools, all were still enrolled although many of the delinquents were dropouts.) The critics claimed that family structure was given undue importance because the vital social status variables had been controlled, and so could not explain delinquent vs. nondelinquent differences. They argued that if family variables had been allowed to compete with ethnic background, social class, and rural-urban residence, the latter variables would have been shown to be the more important. [Studies by Robins (Study R) and Wilson (1962) have since shown that family type *is* an excellent predictor as compared with demographic characteristics, so the Glueck study was not misleading, but this was not known at the time.]

The critics also pointed out that by choosing control subjects still attending school and free of even unofficial delinquency, the Gluecks had chosen controls who were more virtuous than the average nondelinquent. Thus the study was actually comparing the two extremes of a deviance continuum—children so delinquent they had been institutionalized vs. a "super-normal" group. Since the court considers family type in deciding whether a delinquent requires institutionalization, and since intact and cohesive families are more successful than disorganized families in keeping nondelinquent youth in school, once social status factors had been eliminated by matching, the study could hardly avoid finding a very important role for family structure. This is an example of how the choice of the control group can "set up" the findings of a study ahead of time.

Same-sex siblings are in many ways a nearly ideal control group. They are like index cases with regard to sex, race, socioeconomic status, place of rearing, and family characteristics. The only dimension along which they cannot be precisely matched to the index case is age. Being nearly perfect controls, they neatly illustrate the fact that the better the control group, the more unassailable is the argument that differences in outcome are due to differences in the initial condition, but at the same time, the fewer predictor variables can the researcher pursue. With sibling controls, not only are demographic variables lost to investigation, but so are family environment and genetic variables. Designs using same-sex sibling controls have one other weakness as well—they require selecting index cases who have a sibling of the same sex, and this limits the sample to index cases from at least two-child families and among such cases, biases selection toward large families.

There is one circumstance in which the use of sibling controls has a very special advantage—that is, when the index case and his sibling control are reared in different environments. This is the case when siblings are separated by adoption or when the older sibling is spared the family breakup in early childhood experienced by the younger one. These "natural experiments" provide our best hopes for separating nature from nurture in understanding the contribution of parental impact on children's disorders.

In follow-back studies, it is customary to pick controls from the set of records that provide Time 1 information about the index cases. Either random cases or cases matched to each index child's characteristics are selected. In Lane and Albee's follow-back study (Study L) to learn whether schizophrenics had low IQs premorbidly, siblings were the control group. But in addition, classmates matched for IQ to the schizophrenics and *their* siblings provided a second level control. This allowed showing not only that schizophrenics' premorbid IQs were lower than their siblings, but also that the *correlation* found between normal children and their siblings did not occur between the pre-schizophrenic-sibling pairs.

The purpose of a control group is to provide an estimate for what the measures taken in the index cases *would* have been if the index condition or treatment intervention had not occurred. Even with an ideal group, this estimate will be correct only if the controls' participation in the study has not itself influenced these measurements. This problem does not arise when the data come entirely from linking records created independently of the research enterprise at two time periods, as is typical of follow-back studies. However, in prospective studies where baseline and perhaps interval measures as well are made for control as well as index groups, there is the possibility that the experience of being repeatedly measured can influence the measures evaluating the controls' final status. In studies evaluating the effectiveness of psychotherapy, it has even been suggested that the initial interview before allocation to control or treatment groups may itself constitute psychotherapy, leaving the study without a truly untreated group. The argument becomes more plausible if repeated assessments of control subjects are required rather than only at the beginning and end.

The other difficulty with long-term prospective studies that begin with well-matched controls is that greater demands for cooperation as well as greater rewards in terms of friendly interest accrue to the index than to the control subjects, leading to differential dropout rates and thus to progressively poorer matching between index and control groups as time goes by.

A number of strategies can help mitigate these problems of prospective controlled studies, although they do not solve them. If control as well as index cases are chosen only from people who have volunteered to participate as index subjects, there is less likely to be an initial difference in interest and cooperativeness between the two groups—although it might be argued that those who volunteered for treatment but were denied it have been *damaged* by the disappointment, biasing outcomes in favor of the treated group. A second strategy, when repeated measures are deemed necessary, is to divide the control group into subgroups, which are then given different levels of frequency of evaluation: perhaps half evaluated as often as the treated group, the other half evaluated only at the beginning and end. The division should be made so that baseline measures of the subgroups are equal. Then if final measures show equality between the control subgroups, this provides reasonable assurance that repeated measurement has not muddied the final index-control comparison.

Should Control Groups be Problem-Free?—One issue that repeatedly appears with reference to the selection of control groups is whether or not to exclude affected children. Should outcomes of children with behavior problems be compared with outcomes of a general sample of children of similar backgrounds or with outcomes of children with similar backgrounds but free of problems? Eliminating affected children from the control group can be expected to increase the size of differences found, and thus make it possible to find significant differences with smaller samples. However, the screening out of affected children sacrifices an important contribution that a control group can make, in addition to informing us as to whether the index group has different outcomes or predictors: i.e., the controls can provide normative data for the reference population as a whole.

Another important contribution of a control group unselected with respect to the index problem would also be sacrificed: the opportunity to replicate the results found for the index cases. If the subsample of affected cases in the control group differs from the unaffected control cases in the same ways that the index group differs from the total control group, this is powerful support for the findings.

These advantages of an unscreened control group seem to outweigh the statistical advantage of screening. Since the number of affected cases is likely to be small in any case, unless the problems for which index children were selected are common ones, there is not likely to be sufficient benefit to balance the costs. Further, one can always later exclude from calculations those control cases found to have the disorder to see whether differences not significant when comparing index cases with the total control group become significant after the control sample is "purified." Some later "purification" may be necessary to get an unaffected control group even when it has been screened for affected cases initially, since the researcher may discover previously unsuspected affected cases among the controls in the course of the research. For all these reasons, a control sample unselected for the index problem is generally preferable to attempting to obtain a "healthy" control sample.

In follow-up studies that evaluate treatment, an additional problem in interpreting index case vs. control differences arises out of what has been called the "placebo" or "Hawthorne" effect. The observation that receiving a placebo or sham treatment often is associated with improvement has led some scientists to sneer at placebo-responders as overly suggestible or perhaps not having had anything wrong in the first place. This is an unjustified view. Placebo response merely shows that treatment may have nonspecific as well as specific effects. It is reassuring to the child and his family to believe that a professional is taking action about their problem. This reassurance may lead to their undertaking helpful procedures on their own which they had been too demoralized to think of or act on previously. However, the problem usually addressed in treatment evaluation is whether a *particular* treatment is helpful, not whether entry into treatment of *some* kind might be a good idea. Therefore, it is advisable to try to eliminate or compensate for placebo effects.

There are two ways of doing so. First, before beginning the

controlled study, one can subject all index and control subjects to a placebo period, and then drop from the study all who improve so much that they no longer meet entrance criteria. Second, one can provide a treatment program for the control group of a different type, rather than using a treatment-no treatment design. Miller and Dyer's study of Head Start nursery schools is an example of a well-executed study of this kind (Study O), where the controls included not only untreated children but those experiencing a variety of nursery school experiences.

Number of Control Subjects and Matching—If the population of available index cases is small, it is usually desirable to take all available index cases into the sample and then to choose more control than index cases to increase the total sample size. If there are ample index cases, and if the index sample is to be analyzed using variables that pertain exclusively to it—variables such as diagnostic category or type or length of treatment—the most economical plan is to take enough index cases to have sizeable subgroups after subdivision and a smaller control group, since the latter can remain undivided in analysis. When the index cases are plentiful and homogeneously defined, the most efficient sample selection is that in which index and control groups are of equal size. When this is the design, a further possibility arises—one-to-one matching of controls to index cases with respect to important analytic variables they share—such as age, socioeconomic status, or IQ. The advantage of one-to-one matching over the matching for variables in the total sample is that the control subjects then not only have the same distribution of characteristics as the index cases, but the correlations between these characteristics are identical in the two groups. Further, one-to-one matching makes possible—in theory—the use of the powerful statistical techniques devised for matched-pair analysis. The latter advantage is somewhat illusory, however. At follow-up, these initially matched pairs will no longer all be intact. There will be cases where one member of the pair has been located and the other has not. Throwing out successfully followed members of the sample because their paired member is missing in order to use these statistical techniques usually appears too high a price to pay in sample size and representativeness.

Data to Collect Initially

The cardinal rules for data collection are that the same level of data be collected for all cases, that it be reliable, and that it be relevant to the hypotheses to be tested. In prospective studies (whether or not they are catch-up studies), there are three types of relevant data to collect at Time 1: descriptors of variables used as criteria for eligibility to enter the sample, identifiers to allow location at follow-up, and predictors. When the study is a follow-up of children with problems, predictors generally include categorizations of the problems itself along dimensions such as duration, age at onset, age at coming to treatment, nature of symptoms, degree of impairment, plus characteristics of the child in areas other than the disorder, areas such as IQ, school success, personality traits, age, race, sex, birth-order position. Finally there are characteristics of the home and social setting, including the date of study to set it in historical perspective, family history of the disorder, type of family structure (broken, intact, foster family, etc.), socioeconomic status, and place of residence. The choice of predictors obviously depends on what hypotheses are to be tested, and whether one is predicting from a child's status at Time 1 to his later outcome, or from the parents' status at Time 1 to the child's at Time 2. In follow-back studies, descriptors of the selection criteria variables, and identifiers are both collected from Time 2 records for index cases, leaving only predictors to be collected from Time 1 records. For follow-back controls, all three types of information are collected from Time 1 records.

In real-time prospective studies, predictor data missing from the roster from which the case was chosen can be supplemented by interviewing or testing at intake into the study. In catch-up prospective studies and follow-back studies, predictors available at Time 1 are limited to what can be found in the records. These studies may try to supplement the Time 1 data by retrospective questions in interviews at Time 2, giving the respondent the Time 1 date and asking him about his situation or experiences prior to that date. Although obtained as part of a follow-up study, these remain retrospective data, subject to all the limitations of recall and rationalization noted above. Nonetheless it is worth getting such retrospective data, at least for those events that are memorable and easy to date. They are valuable not only for supplementing missing information but for correcting misinformation in the records. As an example, in Robins' study of black school boys (Study R2), whether the father was absent from the home before his son reached age 14 was inferred from the name of the guardian on elementary school records. If on any school record, the guardian's name was not masculine or, if masculine, the last name was not the same as the child's, it was assumed the biologic father had been absent. Estimates based on these criteria were found in interview to have been much too low, apparently because the schools often failed to correct their records when the family dissolved after the first record was made on the occasion of the child's school entry.

In catch-up and follow-back studies, Time 1 data typically are obtained from medical records, school records, police records or social-agency records. These can all be used in real-time prospective studies as well. But in addition real-time prospective studies can include personal interviews with, or written questionnaires from, parents or teachers of young children, and directly from older children, as well as psychological and psychophysiological tests, physical examination, and observations in school rooms, at home, or in the researcher's office.

Sources best used and data collected from them should depend obviously on the study's purposes. Often in a real-time prospective study the easiest way to collect the background data needed is by interviewing the mother. The personal interview, given a systematic structured protocol, can be both a reliable and valid data source, contrary to its detractors' opinions. The personal interview's reputation for unreliability seems to stem mainly from the layman's awe of laboratory science, an awe shared even by social scientists engaged in survey research. Compared with the mysteries of urine tests and X rays, the interview appears a commonplace and crude tool. Feinstein (1967) has shown, however, that experts' reliability in reading X rays is much lower than reputed, perhaps less than the reliability of interviews! Another source of doubt stems from the widespread suspicion that subjects lie and interviewers bias responses by the way they ask questions or record answers. Survey methodology research, however, has shown that lying is infrequent when there is privacy, assurance of confidentiality, and assurance that no decisions about treatment or other aspects of the subject's life depend on the answers given (Study R1). It has also been found that the interviewer influences answers to questions about attitudes much more than questions about facts (Sudman and Bradburn, 1974). Life history interviewing, which concentrates on the occurrence or nonoccurrence of specific events, is not much subject to bias by interviewers' attitudes.

It is difficult to measure the validity of interviews comprehensively because they often ask about feelings and events unknown to anyone other than the person interviewed and about other information not easily subject to confirmation or disconfirmation. One measure of validity that has added to skepticism about the value of interviews is the degree of correspondence between interviews and official records. Discrepancies between interview responses and data found in official records have been assumed to show the inaccuracy of the interview. We noted above, however, that official records can also be inaccurate. Those who use them as yardsticks forget that official records themselves may be based on an interview—more often than not conducted by a clerk or a busy doctor asking questions of untested reliability under circumstances that make the respondent well aware that his answers may affect his chances for a job, for parole, for receiving treatment or welfare payments. These are situations that maximize the chance of falsehood.

Length of the Follow-Up Interval

The length of the follow-up is an important design element. An inappropriate choice can produce misleading results. In a study of transmissions from parent to child, the follow-up interval may need to be a full generation. Thus Bohman's (1972) conclusion that "the occurrence of the biological fathers in the registers of crime or abuse of alcohol was not related to the children's adjustment," while accurately reporting the findings of her study of 11-year-olds does not tell us that this relationship may not occur once the adopted-away children enter the age of risk for crime and alcoholism. Studies in which the offspring of criminals are older (Studies D1, R1, R2) do not find such a salutary situation.

The American Head Start program originally was reported as successful because at the end of the brief nursery school program, enrollees showed gains in IQ compared with controls. When those children were followed into public school, however, the differences vanished. Since the goal of the program was to make culturally deprived children more successful in school, doing the evaluation immediately after terminating the project was the wrong choice of follow-up interval.

On the other hand, when the effect of an experience can be expected to be brief or when the purpose of treatment is to make a difficult but self-limited period of distress shorter or less unpleasant, one can miss the effect entirely by extending the follow-up interval too long. Kandel's study of the effect of having a drug-using friend on the initiation into drugs wisely used a follow-up interval of only a few months (Study K). Had the interval been several years, there is a good chance that the effect of friends' drug-use status at Time 1 would have been obscured by changes in the friends' drug use or a shift to new friends.

Other things being equal, the desirable interval of follow-up is the shortest interval which encompasses the period of risk for the outcome in which the study is interested.

Repeated Assessments During the Follow-Up Interval—The opportunity to do repeated assessments during the follow-up interval is available only in prospective real-time studies. When the purpose of the study is to describe developmental processes or to gather information about how soon to expect treatment effects and what is optimum treatment duration, repeated assessments appear to be the only way to obtain the requisite data. The usual technique is to repeat the same protocol at specified intervals.

When the study requires it, repeated measures can be an elegant research tool. An example is the Jessors' yearly evaluation of how many children had begun a number of socially disapproved behaviors (sex relations, drinking, smoking marijuana) in the previous year (Study J). Without the yearly follow-up, it would not have been possible to show that each year and at each age level the transition probabilities could be predicted from events in the preceding year.

Many studies where the goals do not seem to require interval measurements have nonetheless obtained them. This apparently unnecessary effort often results from the lack of clear commitment at the outset from the researchers, their funding organization, or both as to how long the follow-up would continue. Each data collection point was possibly the final one. An example is the early Glueck follow-up (1940) of delinquents which had three "final" data collections of police records that could have been done once at the end.

An argument offered in favor of repeated measures, even when all necessary data could be obtained at the study's end, has been that keeping in touch with the subjects during the interval enhances the chances of finding them for interview at the final follow-up. This argument is based on a somewhat exaggerated idea of the difficulties in locating subjects after long intervals. Both in countries with and without national registers, it has been found possible to locate almost every case even after long intervals without contact *if* sufficient identifiers have been obtained at Time 1. Even in the United States, a country with a high level of geographic mobility and no population register, follow-up studies have been able to locate more than 90% of samples after intervals of as much as 30 years (Studies R1 and 2). In Sweden, where registers are available, 98% follow-ups after 10- and 15-year intervals have been achieved (Hagnell, 1966).

If the only data to be collected at follow-up come from records, one would suppose that interval assessments should not be necessary, since records made at any time during the interval should be still available at final follow-up in the archives of the police, hospitals, etc. In the last few years, however, in the interests both of saving space and in preserving privacy, there has been a growing practice of destroying records as soon as they become inactive, a practice of great concern to both the researcher and the historian. This destruction is particularly common for records that furnish the best evidence of children's deviance—Juvenile Court records. When records are routinely destroyed, there are indeed good reasons for record monitoring throughout the follow-up interval, rather than only at the termination point.

When the purpose of a follow-up study is to show the effect of parental behavior on children's behavior or symptoms, the follow-up interval should in theory be very brief, since an immediate reaction to the parents can be expected. In fact, the ideal interval is probably *so* brief that the follow-up study is not a practical tool for investigating parental effects on children's behavior. We would like, for instance, to learn whether rejection by the parent incites the child to hostility. To test this, we need index families to follow in which at Time 1 there was a rejecting parent and a child who was *not* hostile, and control families without rejecting parents in which the child was also not hostile. If at follow-up (Time 2), we find that children with rejecting parents have more often become hostile than control children, we would have evidence that parents' rejection does cause hostility. What we are much more likely to find, however, is that our index cases will *still* not be hostile at Time 2, since they have already shown an ability to put up with a rejecting parent amicably at Time 1. We would still not know whether in the great majority of families in which both rejecting parents and hostile children occur, the parents' behavior caused the child's. In our control families, by Time 2, there would probably have appeared some cases in which parents had become rejecting and children had become hostile, but in these cases too we would not know which came first—the parent's behavior or the child's attitude. Rutter (Study T1) points out the inability of his Isle of Wight study to demonstrate such relationships. We must depend on experiments, not follow-up studies of the natural history type, to explore causal relationships between events that normally occur in close temporal proximity.

Outcome Measures

Like the data gathered to describe Time 1, data at the conclusion of a follow-up can be entirely based on records, such as the fact of a psychiatric hospitalization, the number of adult arrests, school achievement test scores, dishonorable discharges from the military, or appearance on welfare rolls; or they can be based on personal interview, psychological tests, questionnaires, or any combination of these with records.

A combination of interview with records is often a profitable one. In the course of attempting to locate respondents after a long interval, one may need to use records as a source of recent addresses. As long as the researcher has to check police or hospital records to locate the subjects, he can include their appearance in these records as part of his outcome criteria at negligible cost.

It is not a negligible cost to go in the opposite direction—to add interviews as outcome data when records alone would appear sufficient. It is dangerous, however, to rely on records alone for judging outcome. In interview, the subject has the opportunity to say either "yes" or "no" to every question. In record searches, only the "yeses" are definite. The researcher is forced to assume both that the records he failed to find did not exist *and* that the subject was at risk of having such a record. Not finding a record, however, is not proof that there is none. The record may be misfiled, the name misspelled, or the name changed. The respondent may not be at risk of having the record in question because, unknown to the researcher, he has emigrated or died or been continuously institutionalized during the follow-up interval. If an attempt is made to interview the respondent as well as check his records, one learns of institutionalizations, deaths, and emigrations, and in interview one can ask questions that reveal whether there ought to be a record for him and under what name. Knowing that a record *should* exist leads to a more intensive search and often success. Thus, in Study R2, interviews indicating men *had* been in military service and *had* finished high school led to renewed and often successful efforts to find these records. A return to search for missing records after interview substantially reduced what would otherwise have appeared to be lying in interview.

Interviewing subjects may seem unnecessary in follow-back studies. After all, the appearance in a particular record source constitutes both the outcome criterion and the criterion for inclusion as an index case. Since the outcome determined the choice of the case, should it be subject to revision by interviewing? Interviewing in follow-back studies has two advantages: it can help the researcher locate the appropriate early records by obtaining childhood addresses, siblings' names, schools attended, and early treatment history, just as it does in prospective studies. Second, it allows the application of more precise criteria for eligibility. Take as an example, Lane and Albee's study of schizophrenia as related to school IQ scores (Study L). They found that schizophrenics in general had lower IQs than their siblings but that those with symptoms of "turning against the self" did not. Since it is well known that psychiatric diagnosis in most hospitals is a very unreliable procedure, it seems likely, given the U.K.-U.S. study showing the overdiagnosis of schizophrenia and underdiagnosis of depression in American hospitals (Cooper, 1970), that many of these cases with "turning against themselves" as a symptom would not have met research criteria for schizophrenia had they been systematically interviewed. Their inclusion may have led to an underestimation of the true association of low IQ with schizophrenia.

Problems of Case Loss

While prospective studies are particularly susceptible to case loss, it can be a serious problem in follow-back studies as well. Follow-back studies can be biased by selectively failing to locate some cases in early records. It is often difficult to tell in reports of follow-back studies how much sample loss has occurred, because the *selection* criteria are often stated as simultaneous appearance in records of both time periods. If there were Time 2 interviews, as suggested above, sample loss could be estimated because the researcher would know whether to *expect* to find the case in the early (Time 1) records.

The chief protection against case loss in real-time prospective studies is foresight—asking at Time 1 for ample identifying information, including birth dates of the subject himself, and parents' and siblings' names and birth dates as well so that if the subject himself is difficult to locate in the future, at least some relative likely to know his address is locatable. It is also advisable at Time 1 to request written permission from the subject or his parents to search records that can help in later location: school records, police records, vital statistics, tax rolls, or registers.

In "catch-up" prospective studies and follow-back studies, one must depend on data collected for other purposes, which may be both inaccurate and incomplete. It is wise to choose the agency whose records will form the population being sampled on the basis of the quality of the records that will furnish the identifiers. Not only should these data be accurate and plentiful, but they should have been collected at *first* contact with the individuals listed. Otherwise, there will be more identifying data for those who have had most treatment, most welfare payments, attended the school longest, or had most arrests. If those receiving most services have most identifiers, they will be easiest to locate and therefore overrepresented at follow-up. When they are compared with a control group, the agency may appear to have had more effect for good or ill than it really has had.

In the United States, concerns about privacy and decreasing reverence for the medical profession and science in general have combined to reduce research interview acceptance rates. The understandable concern that high refusal rates may mean inaccurate results has even led to talk of abandoning survey methods of evaluation. Fortunately, most studies of the effects of sample loss show that refusals do *not* tend to be biased toward either good or poor adjustment as indicated by available record indices. The same cannot be said, however, for losses due to failure to locate cases. Those with extremely poor outcomes—i.e., who die, or go to jail, or to hospitals—are easy to locate, but among the noninstitutionalized survivors, the well-adjusted are generally easier to find than others, because they have more stable residences and maintain contact with relatives.

The relative nonavailability of cases with more deviant adjustments is a problem not only in evaluation at follow-up but also in case selection at Time 1. As Kandel (Study K) showed, children not in school on the day on which baseline measures of drug use were taken were disproportionately heavy users. She found this effect again at Time 2: those who had been present at Time 1 but were not in the classroom on the day of follow-up had been heavier users at Time 1 than those still available. Baltes et al. (1971) similarly found that adolescents available at school for a repeat of an IQ test had higher scores on the original test than had adolescents present only on the first occasion.

Case loss may not be a serious matter in studies of predictors of change. If there are strong relationships between predictor and outcome in the total sample, they will appear even if the sample has become somewhat biased by selective case loss. For studies attempting to obtain accurate estimates of the true prevalence of problems, however, case loss inevitably creates errors. There appears to be no statistical adjustment that can compensate adequately for these lost cases. The best strategy is to lay the groundwork ahead of time for high recovery rates and then do one's best to avoid losses. Although the effects of the losses on estimates will always be unknown, if their number is small, the two estimates calculated on the assumption first that the missing cases all had good outcomes and second that all had bad outcomes will be close together, and the true rate will be somewhere within that narrow range. In studies requiring multiple data collections during the follow-up interval, it is difficult to follow all cases at *each* contact. The researcher should at least designate *one* data collection occasion as the most crucial one and try to reassess *all* cases on that occasion. The most crucial reassessment will usually be the final one.

The concerns about missing cases apply to control as well as to index cases in longitudinal studies. Allowing substitution for hard-to-find control subjects will result in exaggerating differences in outcomes between index and controls. Like index cases, easier-to-find control subjects are also likely to be more stable.

Analyzing Results

Longitudinal studies clearly have advantages over cross-sectional studies in reaching solid scientific conclusions about the way in which a child's own characteristics or his background at one point in time can affect his later life, about early childhood traits that are durable over time as compared with those that are short-lived, and about early indicators of later liability. Yet the accumulation of complicated bodies of data from distinct time periods sometimes presents awesome challenges to the data analyst. The dangers of drawing easy but incorrect conclusions from longitudinal studies have been spelled out eloquently by Campbell and Boruch (1975). They call our attention to two serious problems: first that matching, whether we are matching controls to index cases or matching index cases with one kind of pattern of symptoms to those with a different pattern, is never fully successful. Matching is attempted for those background factors thought likely to have made some contribution both to the occurrence of the index case and to the final outcome. As an example, assuming poverty in childhood contributes both to delinquency and to adult crime rates, when we want to learn the effect of delinquency on later criminality, we match control cases to index cases on poverty level in childhood in order to be able to conclude that differences in outcome are delinquency rather than poverty effects. Not content with poverty alone, we may match as well on other background factors—criminal parents, overcrowding, large sibships—until the controls are, insofar as we can tell, from identical settings as the delinquents. If these background factors are powerful predictors, when all occur together the rate of delinquency in children from such a background may be very high—perhaps over 80%. When we look for a nondelinquent "match" from the same highly delinquigenic background, we either find a "super-child," whose unusual strengths have protected him from responding to these background factors in the usual way, or more probably, we settle for a match less good than we would like. Even when we appear to obtain perfect matches, defined as falling into all the same background categories as our index cases, our matches are probably still imperfect. Take poverty again. To match on this variable, we define a category as "less than X units of income per month" and call those in it as living "in poverty." If poverty and delinquency are in fact related in the real world, we will find the mean earnings of delinquents' families within the poverty category lower than the mean earnings of the nondelinquent control families in the same category. The controls will be clustered just below our upper limit like goldfish feeding at the surface. We can improve the matching by dividing income into finer categories, but the pressure to reestablish the "natural order" will always be exerting itself, within any categories we define.

Campbell's other warning (Campbell and Erlebacher, 1970) is that because all measurements are subject to error, all follow-up studies are biased by regressions to the mean. The argument is that low initial values are more likely to be the products of errors in the low direction, while middle initial values are equally likely to be the products of errors in either direction, and high values are more likely to be the products of errors in the high direction. As a result, at Time 2, there will be "improvement" in low IQ or reading scores or in high symptom scores just by chance. Since we often are interested in changes only in children who begin at the "problem" end of the scale, we fail to notice that the "utterly healthy" have moved toward the mean about as much as the "sick" have improved. We are thus in danger of reading improvement into our results and interpreting any treatment as successful even when it made no difference. Preventing this error is one of the most important functions of control groups.

Stimulated by these caveats, there has been a great ferment in recent years among statisticians in developing methods for handling the statistical analysis of change in ways that can simultaneously control on a variety of predictor variables and assess the net contribution of each when all other factors are held constant. The newest developments also allow measurement errors to be taken into account. This is not an appropriate place (nor am I qualified) to explain these developments in detail. But the serious reader is referred to work by Jöreskog and Sörbom (1976), Heise (1970), and Goodman (1970). While these new methods are mathematically elegant, they usually require large samples and interval measures that our crude, clinical assessments simply cannot provide.

Actuarial statisticians have developed widely used techniques for demonstrating the effects of predictors such as marital status and prior illness on life expectancy. These techniques can be applied to all sorts of outcomes other than death. While not elegant mathematically, they are appropriate for cruder data and they do handle the problems of the amount of the risk period through which cases have passed. Those interested in applying actuarial methods to life history data are referred to Tietze (1968), Rosenberg (1962), and Robins and Wish (1977).

While it is well to consider the new statistical techniques being developed for analyzing data collected at more than one point in time, there remain traditional satisfactory ways of presenting longitudinal data. The most common begin with the classic 2 x 2 contingency table evaluated by χ^2, which compares a single outcome or predictor for two independent samples. After each outcome or predictor has been looked at one at a time, those significantly distinguishing the two groups are allowed to compete in some form of multivariate analysis.

Difficulties in following this simple analytic program occur when the categorization of the data has not been settled before data collection begins. Some of the early real-time prospective studies (e.g., Studies A and E) collected their data *via* diverse methodologies (observations of play, psychological tests, free interviews, school records, physical examinations) and at many time periods. For these studies, before any analysis could proceed, judges had to read the whole collection of many years of observation, interviews with mothers, tests, etc., and transform them impressionistically into rankings. The result is that the final ranks have no clear operational definitions. When Kagan (Study E) reports that aggression is the most stable personality trait, it is not clear that the aggression scored in a 3-year-old is really the same trait as what is called aggression in adults aged 18 to 30.

With the advent of computers, the sensitive judge trying to absorb the total record is no longer necessary. It is now possible to enter data into the computer in detailed fashion and use computer programs to summarize it. An interesting example using factor analysis for this purpose appears in Study M. This study has summarized children's symptoms into empirically based patterns that can be used as diagnostic syndromes.

Notes on Studies[1]

A. Berkeley Growth Study

Study Type: Real-time prospective. *Index Cases:* Subjects were drawn from two initially distinct studies: (1) the Berkeley Guidance Study, which selected healthy full-term babies born in Berkeley over an 18-month period (N = 248) and assigned matched pairs as treatment or control subjects; and (2) the Oakland Growth Study, which selected fifth-graders from five Oakland elementary schools (N = 212). *Length of Follow-Up Interval:* For the Guidance Study sample information was recorded from birth to approximately age 30 years, and for the Oakland Growth Study from fifth grade to approximately 37 years. Many interim studies used shorter intervals. *Interval Measurement:* Semi-annual in the Growth Study and at least yearly to age 14 in the Guidance Study, but with widely fluctuating numbers of cases contacted at different ages. *Data Sources:* Teacher ratings; interviews with subjects, teachers, parents, siblings, spouses; physical assessments; psychological tests; observations of child's behavior; school report cards; sociometric ratings by schoolmates. *Case Recovery:* Varied widely from study to study. Block, and Stewart and Livson both used both samples: Block studying 171 (51%) out of a target group of 336, defined as the treated members of the Guidance Study plus the Oakland Growth Study; Stewart and Livson studying 165 (36%) out of 460. Livson and Peskin, Tuddenham, and Elder all used the Oakland Growth Study only, obtaining data on 30, 34, and 43% respectively. At recovery, spouse and offspring were evaluated as well as the subject himself. *Principal Variables: Time 1:* Characteristics of the family environment (values, democracy, participation) and of the parents (competence, warmth, harmony) for the early studies; children's personality traits, intelligence, school achievement, and economic privation for studies of adults. *Time 2:* Personality types, intelligence, personality, smoking, occupation, general adjustment, behavior, IQ, body build of subject's offspring.

References: Block (1971), Bronson et al. (1959), Elder (1974), Hunt and Eichorn (1972), Livson and Peskin (1967), MacFarlane (1964), Stewart and Livson (1966), Stewart (1962), Tuddenham (1959).

B. Borland: Hyperactive Boys

Study Type: Catch-up prospective. *Index Cases:* 37 white males were selected from old child guidance clinic records if they met five criteria: (1) symptoms satisfied criteria for the hyperactive syndrome, (2) each had a brother, (3) aged 4 to 11 at referral, (4) IQ of 80 +, (5) no physical or medical problems. *Control Cases:* Same-sexed siblings. Substituted brothers-in-law in two cases. *Length of Follow-Up Interval:* 20 to 25 years. *Interval Measurement:* None. *Data Sources:* Clinic records; family physicians; school records, including grades and IQ scores; and interviews. *Case Recovery:* Interviews with 20 index cases (49%) and 19 controls. *Principle*

Variables: Time 1: Number of symptoms of hyperactivity, IQ, school achievement. *Time 2:* Adult symptoms of hyperactivity, school success, socioeconomic situation, hyperactivity in offspring.

Reference: Borland and Heckman (1976).

C. Cambridge-Somerville Youth Study

Study Type: Real-time prospective. *Index Cases:* One boy randomly chosen from each of 253 pairs matched on age (5 to 13), delinquency-proneness, family background and home environment. Pool of subjects came from agency and school recommendations of difficult and average boys in the community. *Control Cases:* The 253 boys *not* selected as index cases. *Length of Follow-Up Interval:* 35 years. *Interval Measurement:* 200 interviewed at about age 23; records searched when they were 31. *Data Sources:* Police, mental hospitals, alcohol treatment centers, questionnaires. *Case Recovery:* 477 located out of 506 (94%). Questionnaire information on 222 (44%): interviewing still in progress. *Principal Variables: Time 1:* Family type, child's delinquency, treatment. *Time 2:* Alcoholism, adult criminal behavior.

References: McCord (1976a and 1976b), McCord and McCord (1959), McCord et al. (1960), Powers and Witmer (1951).

D (1). Danish Adoption Studies: Criminality

Study Type: Catch-up prospective. *Index Cases: Part 1:* 1145 male adoptees born 1927 to 1941. *Part 2:* 143 criminal adoptees whose biological fathers were born since 1890. *Control Cases: Part 1:* 1145 nonadoptees matched on age, sex, occupational status of father, and residence. *Part 2:* 143 adoptees not known to the police, matched for age and adoptive father's occupation. *Length of Follow-Up Interval:* Birth to age 30 to 44 years. *Interval Measurement:* None. *Data Sources:* Adoption records, police records, psychiatric register, midwives' reports. *Case Recovery:* Information obtained on 971 biological fathers of 1145 adoptees (85%) and on 1120 fathers of 1145 nonadoptees (98%). *Principle Variables: Time 1:* Criminal status of biological and adoptive parents. *Time 2:* Criminal record of adoptees vs. nonadoptees. Psychiatric diagnoses of biological parents of criminal and non-criminal adoptees.

Reference: Hutchings and Mednick (1975).

D (2). Danish Adoption Studies: Schizophrenia

Study Type: Catch-up prospective. *Index Cases:* 173 biological and 74 adoptive relatives of 34 persons adopted between 1924 and 1947 and unanimously classified as schizophrenic by four researchers on the basis of abstracts of mental hospital records (out of 507 hospitalized). *Control Cases:* 174 biological relatives and 91 adoptive relatives of 34 adoptees who had never lived in a mental institution, matched on age, sex, socioeconomic status of rearing family, time spent with biological relatives, in child care or in foster home before transfer to adoptive home. *Length of Follow-Up Interval:* From 30 to 50 years. *Interval Measurement:* None. *Data Sources:* Institutional records, interviews. *Case Recovery:* Interviews with 329 of 512 relatives (64%). *Principal Variables: Time 1:* Sex and kinship to index or control case. *Time 2:* Psychiatric diagnosis.

Reference: Kety et al. (1968, 1975).

E. Fels Research Institute Study

Study Type: Real-time prospective study. *Index Cases:* 300 newborns. 6–15 added each year since 1929. *Length of Follow-Up Interval:* 19–29 years. *Interval Measurement:* Frequent assessment through age 10. Semi-annual home visits and observations in school and camp settings: biannual interviews in adolescence. *Data Sources:* Behavioral observations, physical growth measurements. IQ and achievement tests, projective tests, parent ratings, interviews with mother and child. *Case Recovery:* Kagan and Moss (1960) studied 54 subjects born between 1930 and 1939, 36 percent of those entering the sample in those years. Kagan and Freeman studied 50 subjects. Moss and Kagan (1961) studied 71 subjects aged 20–29. *Principal Variables: Time 1:* IQ, socioeconomic status, early personality traits, maternal rearing patterns. *Time 2:* adolescent and adult personality (achievement, aggression, sexuality, passivity, dependence, anxiety, etc.) and intelligence.

References: Kagan and Freeman (1963), Kagan and Moss (1960, 1962), Moss and Kagan (1961).

F. Forssman and Thuwe: Refused Abortions

Study Type: Catch-up prospective. *Index Cases:* 120 children surviving to age 21 out of pregnancies which went to term after the mother requested and was refused an abortion. Applications for abortion were during 1939–1941 in Göteborg. *Control Cases:* The next same-sexed child born in the same hospital and surviving (N=119). *Length of Follow-Up Interval:* Birth to age 21. *Interval Measurement:* None. *Data Sources:* Registry offices, child welfare boards, school records, hospitals, guidance clinics, mental hospitals, penal register, military, temperance boards. *Case Recovery:* All were located in records. *Principal Variables: Time 1:* Maternal age, socioeconomic status, broken home. *Time 2:* Psychiatric treatment, alcoholism, education, military service, delinquency, marital status, receipt of public assistance.

Reference: Forssman and Thuwe (1966).

G. Glueck: Delinquent Boys

Study Type: Real-time prospective. *Index Cases:* 500 white males committed to a correctional school. *Control Cases:* 500 schoolboys free of both official and unofficial delinquency matched by residence, age, ethnicity, global IQ. *Length of Follow-Up Interval:* 15 to 22 years: Boys aged 9 to 17 at intake were followed at age 31. *Interval Measurement:* At age 25. *Data Sources:* Criminal data from police and court sources: interviews with subject, parents, wife, others; records of settlement houses, boys' clubs, family welfare agencies. *Case Recovery:* 463 delinquents and 466 nondelinquents at age 25 (83%), 438 delinquents and 442 nondelinquents at age 31 (88%). *Principal Variables: Time 1:* Seriousness of offense history. *Time 2:* Educational attainment, marital stability, criminality, mobility, health, psychiatric care, occupational attainment, leisure interests, military history.

Reference: Glueck and Glueck (1968).

H. Havighurst: River City

Study Type: Real-time follow-up. *Index Cases:* 487 children aged eleven. *Length of Follow-Up Interval:* nine years (to age 20). *Interval Measurement:* Tested from sixth through twelfth grades. *Data Sources:* Intelligence tests; ratings by teachers; sociometric tests; talent tests; psychological tests; interviews with subject, employers, college counselors; court records. *Case Recovery:* Most of the analyses of adult adjustment are limited to 411 individuals (84%). *Principal Variables: Time 1:* IQ, leadership, talent, personal and social adjustment, social class. *Time 2:* school progress, including college attendance; early marriage; work adjustment; competence (work history, adjustment in college, marital history, criminal behavior).

Reference: Havighurst et al. (1962).

I. Heber: Children of Mothers with Low IQs

Study Type: Real-time prospective. *Index Cases:* Half of 40 infants born to mothers with IQs less than 70 in an urban poverty area, randomly assigned to treatment of mother and child. *Control Cases:* (a) half of 40 infants born to mothers with IQs less than 70 randomly assigned to control status, (b) siblings of treatment and control cases. *Length of Follow-Up Interval:* Birth to age 7. *Interval Measurement:* Very frequent (every three weeks). *Data Sources:* IQ tests, tests of language development. *Case Recovery:* All recovered. *Principal Variables: Time 1:* Mother's IQ, infant's IQ. *Time 2:* Children's IQ and language development, mother-child interaction, speech patterns.

References: Heber (1971), Heber and Garber (1974).

J. Jessors: Colorado Students

Study Type: Real-time prospective. *Index Cases:* A random stratified sample of 1126 students from three junior high schools, 2220 from three high schools and 497 from a college. *Length of Follow-Up Interval:* Four years for most items. *Interval Measurement:* Yearly questionnaire administration. *Data Sources:* Questionnaires given to subjects in groups. *Case Recovery:* Four years' data available on 432 (30%) of junior high sample, 205 (41%) of college sample. Two years' information available on 692 (31%) of the students in the high school sample. *Principal Variables: Time 1:* Personal values: perceptions; beliefs; conventionality; history of drinking, sexual experience, marijuana use; deviance; church attendance; grade point average. *Time 2:* Year of transition to drinking, marijuana use, nonvirginity; attitudes toward parents and peers.

References: Jessor (1976), Jessor and Jessor (1975a, 1975b); Jessor et al. (1973).

K. Kandel: New York State High School Students

Study Type: Real-time prospective. *Index Cases:* 10130 New York State public secondary school students. *Length of Follow-Up Interval:* five to six months. *Interval Measurement:* None. *Data Sources:* Questionnaires to students and parents. *Case Recovery:* 5468 (54%) with Time 2 questionnaires that could be matched to Time 1 questionnaire. *Principal Variables: Time 1:* Amount and type of drug use, parents' drug use, best friend's drug use, attitudes toward drug use, year in high school, ethnicity. *Time 2:* Amount and type of drug use.

References: Kandel (1975a and 1975b), Kandel et al. (1976).

L. Lane and Albee: IQs of Schizophrenics

Study Type: Follow-back. *Index Cases:* 36 schizophrenics in state and Veterans Administration hospitals who had no sign of childhood schizophrenia and had school test information available for themselves and a sibling; spouses and children of schizophrenics who attended the same schools. *Control Cases:* 35 cases matched on IQ score in second grade (age seven) identified in school records. Control had to have a sibling with an available IQ score. *Length of Follow-Up Measurement:* Second grade to adult. Maximum interval approximately 24 years. *Interval Measurement:* None. *Data Sources:* School and hospital records. *Case Recovery:* Unknown. Cases admitted only if recoverable. *Principal Variables: Time 1:* IQ scores of schizophrenics, matched controls, and siblings in second grade. *Time 2:* Adult psychiatric status, IQs in records of the same school district for children and spouses of schizophrenics.

References: Lane and Albee (1964, 1965, 1968), Lane et al. (1970).

M. Langner: Manhattan Child Follow-Up

Study Type: Real-time prospective. *Index Cases:* 1034 children aged six to 18, a representative sample of Manhattan (New York City) children. *Length of Follow-Up Interval:* Five years. *Interval Measurement:* None. *Data Sources:* Interviews with mothers and children. *Case Recovery:* 732 cases (71%). *Principal Variables: Time 1:* Stressful life events (illness, change in economic well-being in the household); behavior patterns (dependence, fighting, conflict, isolation, weak group membership); family functioning; race. *Time 2:* Disturbed behavior patterns; behavioral stability and change.

References: Gersten et al. (1976), Langner et al. (1976).

N. Mednick and Schulsinger: Children of Schizophrenic Mothers

Study Type: Real-time prospective. *Index Cases:* 207 children of schizophrenic mothers, with median age of 15. *Control Cases:* 104 subjects with no known mental illness in parents or grandparents matched for age, sex, social class, years of education, placement out of parental home, rural-urban residence. *Length of Follow-Up Measurement:* Eight to 12 years (so far). Follow-up at ages 18 to 30. *Interval Measurement:* Interview and check of psychiatric register after four years. *Data Sources:* Clinical interviews; psychophysiological assessments; psychiatric and psychological examinations; interviews on life history and school behavior; parent interviews, school reports, midwife's report; check of psychiatric register for child, parents, and other relatives; mother's hospital records. *Case Recovery:* 173 of 207 high-risk subjects; 91 of 104 low-risk subjects. *Principal Variables: Time 1:* Psychophysiological status, psychiatric problems, mother's premorbid history, severity of mother's illness, contact with mother and father, perinatal complications. *Time 2:* Current diagnostic status.

References: Mednick (1973), Mednick (1970), Schulsinger (1976).

O. Miller and Dyer: Preschool Programs

Study Type: Real-time prospective. *Index Cases:* From the pool of those who registered for Head Start classes in four areas of Louisville, Kentucky, students were randomly selected and assigned to one of four experimental Head Start nursery school programs: Bereiter-Engelmann; Darcee; Montessori; and Traditional. By the end of the prekindergarten years the total in experimental classes was 214. *Control Cases:* Two control samples: (1) 34 children, 22 drawn from waiting lists for Head Start and 12 from names supplied by the teachers and principals, often preschool brothers and sisters of children enrolled in the school. (2) 15 low-income children who had not attended Head Start, but had entered special kindergarten classes using behavior modification principles. *Length of Follow-Up Interval:* Four years, except for the second control group which had three years. *Interval Measurement:* Assessment of the four treatment modalities to demonstrate their difference; psychological tests, behavioral inventories. *Data Sources:* Tests and rating scales on subjects; information forms filled out by parents. *Case Recovery:* 175 of 214 experimental cases; 29 of 34 Control Group 1 cases; 11 of 15 Control Group 2 cases. *Principal Variables: Time 1:* Prekindergarten IQ; program type, sex. *Time 2:* Achievement, IQ, behavior.

Reference: Miller and Dyer (1975).

P. National Child Development Study

Study Type: Catch-up prospective. *Index Cases:* 17418 children comprising a one-week birth cohort in England, Wales and Scotland in March 1958, originally studied in a survey of the causes of perinatal death. *Length of Follow-Up Interval:* Birth to eight years. *Interval Measurement:* These are interval studies. Children were followed at age seven. There is a still unpublished follow-up at age eleven. *Data Sources:* At birth: obstetric, sociological, and medical information. At age seven: teachers' reports, achievement and psychological tests, medical examination, interviews with biological or adoptive parents, records of adoption. *Case Recovery:* 15468 in follow-up (89%). For study of illegitimate births, 526 of 679 followed up (77%). For study of adopted children, 145 of 205 interviews with adoptive parents (71%). *Principal Variables: Time 1:*

Obstetric factors, illegitimacy, adoptive status, sex, class, home characteristics. *Time 2:* School achievement, adjustment, intelligence, physical development.

References: Crellin et al. (1971), Davie et al. (1972), Seglow et al. (1972).

Q. The National Survey of Health and Development

Study Type: Real-time prospective. *Index Cases:* A birth cohort of 5362 individuals born in Great Britain the first week of March, 1946. *Control Cases:* A subgroup was excluded from tests to provide a comparison with those given repeated evaluations. *Length of Follow-Up Interval:* Birth to thirties. *Interval Measurement:* IQ tests at ages 8, 11, and 15. Teacher ratings at ages 13 and 15; self-rating psychological inventory at 13. School physical examinations at ages 6, 7, 11, and 15; parent questionnaires at ages 4, 6, 8, 9, 11, and 15. *Data Sources:* Teachers, parents, doctors, employment offices, police and court records, school achievement records, examinations, questionnaires completed by survey member, school setting descriptions from school. *Case Recovery:* 77% with full educational test results; 98% have some follow-up information. *Principal Variables: Time 1:* Home environment (insecurity, family breakup, education encouragement), social class, early symptoms of disturbed behavior, hospital admissions. *Time 2:* School attainment, delinquency, enuresis, illegitimacy.

References: Douglas (1964, 1966, 1970, 1975), Douglas et al. (1968), Wadsworth (1976).

R (1). Robins: St. Louis Child Guidance Study

Study Type: Catch-up prospective. *Index Cases:* 503 consecutive white patients with an IQ over 80 seen at a Child Guidance Clinic who survived past age 25. *Control Cases:* 91 subjects with problem-free elementary school records matched on race, age, sex, IQ, and socioeconomic status who survived past age 25. *Length of Follow-Up Interval:* Median age at referral was 13. Interviewed approximately 30 years later. *Interval Measurement:* None. *Data Sources:* Clinic records, police, school, hospital, and many other records. Personal interview. School and police records for their sons. *Case Recovery:* Interviews obtained for 82%; some records for 98%. *Principal Variables: Time 1:* Symptoms in childhood; antisocial and other behavior problems of parents; childhood social status. *Time 2:* Psychiatric diagnosis (in particular, sociopathy), crime, alcoholism, marital stability, mortality, school and police records of offspring.

References: Robins (1974), Robins and O'Neal (1958a and 1958b), Robins and Lewis (1966), Robins et al, (1962a and 1962b).

R (2). Robins: Black School Boys as Adults

Study Type: Catch-up prospective. *Index Cases:* 235 black males born and raised in St. Louis, Missouri, with an IQ of 85 or higher, selected from elementary school records. *Length of Follow-Up Interval:* Approximately 20 years. *Interval Measurement:* None. *Data Sources:* School, police, military and other record sources for men, wives, and children. Interview with subject. *Case Recovery:* Interviews for 223; records for all. *Principal Variables: Time 1:* Home environment, early childhood behavior, school success, juvenile delinquency. *Time 2:* adult psychiatric status, adult deviance (crime, drug abuse, alcoholism), educational and economic outcomes, school success, and delinquency of offspring.

References: Robins (1972), Robins and Hill (1966), Robins and Murphy (1967), Robins and Wish (1977), Robins et al. (1968, 1971, 1975).

S. Roff: Military Service of Child Guidance Cases

Study Type: A. Catch-up prospective; B. Follow-back. *Index Cases:* Cases for which adequate information is available both in military and child guidance clinic records. For catch-up study: 265 delinquents. For follow-back study: 104 with military discharge for psychoneurosis and 164 with discharge for bad conduct. *Control Cases:* For catch-up: randomly chosen school boys. For follow-back: High-ranking enlisted men without discipline problems who had been clinic patients. *Length of Follow-Up Interval:* Approximately eight years. *Interval Measurement:* None. *Data Sources:* Child guidance clinic records; military acceptance or rejection, military discharge, Veterans Administration records; school records. *Case Recovery:* Not reported. *Principal Variables: Time 1:* Childhood maladjustment, personality problems, family background (status, interaction, structure), delinquency, peer relations. *Time 2:* Success in military service.

References: Roff (1960, 1969, 1970, 1972).

T (1). Rutter: Isle of Wight Study

Study Type: Real-time follow-up. *Index Cases:* Isle of Wight—A total school population of 10–11-year-olds (N = 2334). *Control Cases:* A sample of all 10-year-olds in an inner London borough. *Length of Follow-Up Interval:* Four years. *Interval Measurement:* None on the total sample. Some ongoing intervention studies during the interval. *Data Sources:* Tests, teacher and parent questionnaires, medical exams, interviews with children, survey questionnaires to subjects at Time 2. *Case Recovery:* Not clear. *Principal Variables:*

Time 1: Family characteristics; nature and severity of psychiatric, physical, and intellectual-educational problems. *Time 2:* Continued manifestation of problem behaviors.

References: Rutter et al. (1970, 1975, 1976a, and 1976b).

T (2). Rutter and Lockyer: Autistic Children

Study Type: Catch-Up Prospective. *Index Cases:* 64 prepubescent patients with a hospital diagnosis of childhood psychosis or autism. *Control Cases:* 63 nonpsychotic psychiatric patients of the same sex and IQ seen the same year. *Length of Follow-Up Interval:* 12–20 years. *Interval Measurement:* At 9–10 years. *Data Sources:* Hospital records (Time 1); neurological and psychiatric examination, observation, interview with parent, psychological tests (interval evaluation); mail questionnaires to parents and hospital and clinic records (final assessment). *Case Recovery:* All psychotics followed: 61 controls included in the interval evaluation; not followed for the final assessment. *Principal Variables: Time 1:* IQ, presence or absence of speech, neurological signs, response to sound, behavior problems, interpersonal relationships. *Time 2:* Institutionalization, educational level, marriage, occupation, speech, social skills, convulsions, IQ, psychological tests.

References: Lockyer and Rutter (1969), Rutter (1970), Rutter et al. (1967).

U. Terman Study of the Gifted

Study Type: Real-time prospective. *Index Cases:* 1528 children in grades 1 to 12 in California schools who scored in the top 1% on an IQ test. *Control Cases:* 533 unselected subjects given psychological tests. *Length of Follow-Up Interval:* Forty years. *Interval Measurement:* Frequent: 3 field studies 6, 18, and 30 years after entry. Annual reporting by mail in first five years. Mail contact after 14 years, 23 years, 28 years, and 33 years. *Data Sources:* Interviews with family and subject, questionnaires to parents, teachers, subjects. Teachers' observations, medical examinations, school records, school achievement tests, home visits. *Case Recovery:* 1188 replied to 40-year-later Information Blank (74% of total; 85% of survivors), only 2% entirely lost. *Principal Variables: Time 1:* Family values, personality traits and motivation, health, and school progress. *Time 2:* Mortality, health, psychological adjustment, alcohol use, crime, homosexuality, occupation, marital status, fertility, income.

References: Oden (1968), Terman and Oden (1947, 1959).

V. Thomas and Chess: New York Longitudinal Study

Study Type: Real-time prospective. *Index Cases:* 136 children followed from infancy. *Length of Follow-Up Interval:* 16 years (for the 95 older cases). *Interval Measurement:* Frequent during first five years. *Data Sources:* Interviews with parent and child; clinical psychiatric evaluation; behavioral and psychometric data. *Case Recovery:* 90 of 95 who had reached age 16. *Principal Variables: Time 1:* Early personality traits ("temperament"), parent attitudes, early childhood behavior problems. *Time 2:* New behavioral disturbance in adolescence, remission.

References: Thomas and Chess (1976), Thomas et al. (1968).

W. Watt: School Records of Schizophrenics

Study Type: Follow-back. *Index Cases:* 54 schizophrenics aged 15–34 at admission to Massachusetts mental hospitals between 1958 and 1965, who were found to have school records in one town. *Control Cases:* 143 cases drawn from the school records and matched for age, sex, race, father's occupation, and father's education, who had never been in a mental hospital in Massachusetts. Three controls were chosen for most index cases. *Length of Follow-Up Interval:* 10 to 28 years (from school entry to admission to hospital). *Interval Measurement:* None. *Data Sources:* Hospital register, school records. *Case Recovery:* Selection required presence in both Time 1 and Time 2 records. *Principal Variables: Time 1:* Behavior patterns in school (e.g., conscientiousness, assertiveness, conformity); school achievement, IQ. *Time 2:* Adult diagnosis of schizophrenia.

References: Watt et al. (1970, 1976).

Y. Wolfgang: Delinquency in a Cohort

Study Type: Catch-up prospective. *Index Cases:* 9945 boys born in 1945 who lived continuously in Philadelphia from ages 10 to 18, selected from public, parochial, and private schools. *Length of Follow-Up Interval:* Birth to end of juvenile court jurisdiction (age 18). *Interval Measurement:* None. *Data Sources:* School and police records. *Case Recovery:* Not an issue. *Principal Variables: Time 1:* Race, school attended, IQ, achievement level, final grade reached, census tract of last residence (used for social class assignment), physical handicap, residential moves. *Time 2:* Severity of offenses, recidivism, type of crime.

Reference: Wolfgang et al. (1972).

Z. Youth in Transition

Study Type: Real-time prospective. *Index Cases:* 2281 tenth-grade boys (age 15) selected in a multi-stage national sample (1966). *Length of Interval Covered:* Eight years. *Interval Measurement:* Recontacted after 18 months, 30 months, and 42 months. *Data Sources:* Personal interview, tests, questionnaires. Questionnaires for teachers, principals, school counselors. *Case Recovery:* 1365 found for fifth wave (60%). *Principal Variables: Time 1:* Home environment, family size, family values, residence, race, socioeconomic status, academic progress, grades, delinquency, IQ, self-concept, motivation, values. *Time 2:* High school dropout, values and attitudes in high school; enlisting in the military; drug use, smoking, alcohol; delinquency; employment.

References: Bachman (1970), Bachman et al. (1971), Johnston (1973), Johnston and Bachman (1972).

Acknowledgments

This work was supported in part by U.S. National Institutes of Health Grants MH-18864, MH-14677, and DA-00013.

This chapter is an abbreviated version of a chapter published originally in *Grundlagen und Methoden der Psychiatrie*, volume 1. It is reproduced by permission of the publisher, Springer-Verlag (Heidelberg), 1979.

References

[1]This bibliography was prepared with the great assistance of Kathryn Strother Ratcliff, Ph. D.

Bachman, J.G.: Youth in transition, Vol. II: The impact of family background and intelligence on tenth-grade boys. Ann Arbor: Institute for Social Research 1970.

Bachman, J.G., Green, S., Wirtanen, I.D.: Youth in transition, Vol. III: Dropping out—problem or symptom. Ann Arbor: Institute for Social Research 1971.

Baltes, P.B.: Longitudinal and cross-sectional sequences in the study of age and generation effects. Hum. Devel. *11*:145–171 (1968).

Baltes, P.B., Schaie, K.W., Nardi, A.H.: Age and experimental mortality in a seven-year longitudinal study of cognitive behavior. Develop. Psychol. *5*:18–26 (1971).

Baltes, P.B., Nesselroade, J.R., Schaie, K.W., Labouvie, B.W.: On the dilemma of regression effects in examining ability-level-related differentials in ontogenetic patterns of intelligence. Develop. Psychol. *6*:78–84 (1972).

Block, J.: Lives through time. Berkeley: Bancroft Books 1971.

Bohman, M.: A study of adopted children, their background, environment, and adjustment. Acta paediat. scand. *61*:90–97 (1972).

Borland, B.L., Heckman, H.K.: Hyperactive boys and their brothers. Arch. gen. Psychiat. *33*:669–675 (1976).

Bronson, W.C., Katten, E.S., Livson, N.: Patterns of authority and affection in two generations. J. abnorm. soc. Psychol. *58*:143–152 (1959).

Campbell, D.T., Boruch, R.F.: Making the case for randomized assignment to treatments by considering the alternatives. *In:* Evaluation and experiment (C.A. Bennett and A.A. Lumsdaine, Eds.). New York: Academic Press 1975.

Campbell, D.T., Erlebacher, A.E.: How regression artifacts in quasi-experimental evaluations can mistakenly make compensatory education look harmful. *In:* Compensatory education: a national debate, Vol. 3 (J. Hellmuth, Ed.). New York: Brunner/Mazel 1970.

Crellin, E., Kellmer Pringle, M.L., West, P.: Born illegitimate. London: National Foundation for Educational Research in England and Wales 1971.

Davie, R., Butler, N., Goldstein, H.: From birth to seven. London: Longman 1972.

Douglas, J.W.B.: The Home and the School. London: Macgibbon and Kee 1964.

Douglas, J.W.B.: The school progress of nervous and troublesome children. Brit. J. Psychiat. *112*:1115–1116 (1966).

Douglas, J.W.B.: Broken families and child behavior. J. roy. Coll. Physicians Lond. *4*:203–210 (1970).

Douglas, J.W.B.: Early hospital admissions and later disturbances of behaviour and learning. Develop. Med. Child Neurol. *17*:456–480 (1975).

Douglas, J.W.B., Ross, J.M., Simpson, H.R.: All Our Future. London: Peter Davies 1968.

Elder, G.H.: Children of the great depression. Chicago: University of Chicago Press 1974.

Farrington, D.P., Gundry, G., West, D.J.: The familial transmission of criminality. Med. Sci. Law, *15*:177–186 (1975).

Feinstein, A.R.: Clinical judgment. Baltimore, Md: Williams and Wilkins 1967.

Forssman, H., Thuwe, I.: One hundred and twenty children born after application for therapeutic abortion refused. Acta psychiat. scand. *42*:71–88 (1966).

Gersten, J.C., Langner, T.S., Eisenberg, J.G., Simcha-Fagan, O., McCarthy, E.D.: Stability and change in types of behavioral disturbance of children and adolescents. J. abnorm. Child Psychol. *4*:111–127 (1976).

Glueck, S., Glueck, E.: Juvenile delinquents grown up. New York: The Commonwealth Fund 1940.

Glueck, S., Glueck, E.: Delinquents and nondelinquents in perspective. Cambridge: Harvard University Press 1968.

Goodman, L.A.: The multivariate analysis of qualitative data: Interactions among multiple classifications. J. Amer. Statist. Assoc. *65*:225–256 (1970).

Hagnell, O.: A prospective study of the incidence of mental disorder. Stockholm: Scandinavian University Books 1966.

Havighurst, R.J., Bowman, P.H., Liddle, G., Matthews, C., Pierce, J.: Growing up in River City. New York: Wiley 1962.

Heber, R.: Rehabilitation of families at risk for mental retardation: A progress report. Madison, Wisc.: Rehabilitation Research and Retraining Center in Mental Retardation 1971.

Heber, R., Garber, H.: Progress Report III: An experiment in the prevention of cultural-familial retardation. *In:* Proceedings of the Third International Congress of the International Association for the Scientific Study of Mental Deficiency (1974).

Heise, D.R.: Causal inference from panel data. *In:* Sociological methodology (E.F. Borgatta and G.W. Bohrnstedt, Eds.). San Francisco: Jossey-Bass 1970.

Hunt, J.V., Eichorn, D.H.: Maternal and child behaviors: A review of data from the Berkeley Growth Study, Semin. Psychiat. *4*:367–381 (1972).

Hutchings, B., Mednick, S.A.: Registered criminality in the adoptive and biological parents of registered male criminal adoptees. *In:* Genetic Research in Psychiatry

(R. Fieve, D. Rosenthal, and H. Brill, Eds.). Baltimore, Md: Johns Hopkins 1975.

Jessor, R.: Predicting time of onset of marijuana use: A developmental study of high school youth, J. consult. clin. Psychol. 44, *1*:125–134 (1976).

Jessor, R., Jessor, S.L.: Adolescent development and the onset of drinking: A longitudinal study. J. Stud. Alcohol 36, *1*:27–51 (1975a).

Jessor, S.L., Jessor, R.: Transition from virginity to nonvirginity among youth: A social-psychological study over time. Develop. Psychol. 11, *4*:473–484 (1975b).

Jessor, R., Jessor, S.L., Finney, J.: A social psychology of marijuana use: Longitudinal studies of high school and college youth. J. Personal. soc. Psychol. 26, *1*:1–15 (1973).

Johnston, L.: Drugs and American youth. Ann Arbor: Institute for Social Research 1973.

Johnston, J., Bachman, J.G.: Youth in transition Vol. V: Young men and military service. Ann Arbor: Institute for Social Research 1972.

Jöreskog, K.G., Sörbom, D.: Statistical models and methods for analysis of longitudinal data. *In:* Latent variables in socioeconomic models (D.J. Aigner and A.S. Goldberger, Eds.). New York: North-Holland 1976.

Kagan, J., Freeman, M.: Relation of childhood intelligence, maternal behaviors, and social class to behavior during adolescence. Child Develop. *34*:899–911 (1963).

Kagan, J., Moss, H.A.: The stability of passive and dependent behavior from childhood through adulthood. Child Develop. *31*:577–591 (1960).

Kagan, J., Moss, H.A.: Birth to maturity, New York: Wiley 1962.

Kandel, D.: Reaching the hard-to-reach: Illicit drug use among high school absentees. Addictive Diseases 1. *4*:465–480 (1975a).

Kandel, D.: Stages in adolescent involvement in drug use. Science *190*:912–914 (1975b).

Kandel, D., Single, E., Kessler, R.: The epidemiology of drug use among New York State high school students: Distribution, trends, and change in rates of use. Amer. J. publ. Health *66*:43–53 (1976).

Kety, S.S., Rosenthal, D., Wender, P.H., Schulsinger, F.: The types and prevalence of mental illness in the biological and adoptive families of adopted schizophrenics. *In:* The Transmission of Schizophrenia (D. Rosenthal and S.S. Kety, Eds.). Oxford: Pergamon 1968, pp. 345–362.

Kety, S.S., Rosenthal, D., Wender, P.H., Schulsinger, F., Jacobsen, B.: Mental illness in the biological and adoptive families of adopted individuals who have become schizophrenic: A preliminary report based on psychiatric interviews. *In:* Genetic Research in Psychiatry (R. Fieve, D. Rosenthal, and H. Brill, Eds.). Baltimore, Md: Johns Hopkins 1975, pp. 147–165.

Lane, E.A., Albee, G.W.: Early childhood intellectual differences between schizophrenic adults and their siblings. J. abnorm. soc. Psychol. *68*:193–195 (1964).

Lane, E.A., Albee, G.W.: Childhood intellectual differences between schizophrenic adults and their siblings. Amer. J. Orthopsychiat. *35*:747–753 (1965).

Lane, E.A., Albee, G.W.: On childhood intellectual decline of adult schizophrenics: A reassessment of an earlier study, J. abnorm. Psychol. *73*:174–177 (1968).

Lane, E.A., Albee, G.W., Doll, I.S.: The intelligence of children of schizophrenics. Develop. Psychol. 2. *3*:315–317 (1970).

Langner, T.S., Gersten, J.C., McCarthy, E.D., Eisenberg, J.C., Greene, E.L., Herson, J.H., Jameson, J.D.: A screening inventory for assessing psychiatric impairment in children 6 to 18. J. consult. clin. Psychol. 44:286–296 (1976).

Livson, N., Peskin, H.: Prediction of adult psychological health in a longitudinal study. J. abnorm. Psychol. *72*:509–518 (1967).

Lockyer, L., Rutter, M.: A five to fifteen-year follow-up study of infantile psychosis. III: Psychological aspects. Brit. J. Psychiat. *115*:865–882 (1969).

McCord, J.: Patterns of deviance. Paper presented at the Annual Meeting of the Society for Life History Research in Psychopathology (1976a).

McCord, J.: A thirty-year follow-up of treatment effects. Paper presented at the meetings of the American Association of Psychiatric Services for Children (1976b).

McCord, W., McCord, J.: Origins of crime. New York: Columbia University Press 1959.

McCord, W., McCord, J., Gudeman, J.: Origins of alcoholism. Palo Alto: Stanford University Press 1960.

MacFarlane, J.W.: Perspectives on personality and change from the Guidance Study. Vita hum. *7*:115–126 (1964).

Mednick, B.R.: Breakdown in high-risk subjects: Familial and early environmental factors. J. abnorm. Psychol. *82*:469–475 (1973).

Mednick, S.A.: Breakdown in individuals at high risk for schizophrenia: Possible predispositional perinatal factors. Ment. Hygiene *54*:50–63 (1970).

Mednick, S.A., Mura, E., Schulsinger, F., Mednick, B.: Perinatal conditions and infant development in children with schizophrenic parents. Social Biol. *18* (Suppl.). S103–S113 (1971).

Mednick, S.A., Mura, E., Schulsinger, F., Mednick, B.: Erratum and further analysis: "Perinatal conditions and infant development in children with schizophrenic parents." Social Biol. *20*:111–112 (1973).

Miller, L.B., Dyer, J.L.: Four preschool programs: Their dimensions and effects. Monogr. Soc. Res. Child Develop. *40*:1–170 (1975).

Moss, H.A., Kagan, J.: Stability of achievement and recognition seeking behaviors from early childhood through adulthood. J. abnorm. soc. Psychol. *62*:504–513 (1961).

Niswander, K., Gordon, M.: The women and their pregnancies. Philadelphia: Saunders 1972.

Oden, M.H.: The fulfillment of promise: 40 year follow-up of the Terman gifted group. Genet. Psychol. Monogr. *77*:3–93 (1968).

O'Donnell, J.A., Voss, H.L., Clayton, R.R., Slatin, G.T., Room, R.G.: Young men and drugs—a nationwide survey. Rockville, Md: NIDA Research Monograph Ser. 5; DHEW Publ. No. ADM-76-311 (1976).

Powers, E., Witmer, H.: An experiment in the prevention of delinquency. New York: Columbia University Press 1951.

Robins, L.N.: An actuarial evaluation of the causes and consequences of deviant behavior in young black men. *In:* Life history research in psychopathology, Vol. 2 (M. Roff, L.N. Robins, and M. Pollack, Eds.). Minneapolis: University of Minnesota Press 1972, pp. 137–154.

Robins, L.N.: Evaluation of psychiatric services for children in the United States. *In:* Roots of evaluation (J.K. Wing and, H. Hatner, Eds). London: Oxford University Press 1973.

Robins, L.N.: Deviant children grown up. Huntington, N.Y.: Krieger 1974, rev. ed.

Robins, L.N., Hill, S.Y.: Assessing the contributions of family structure, class and peer groups to juvenile delinquency, J. crim. Law Criminal Police Sci. *57*:325–334 (1966).

Robins, L.N., Lewis, R.G.: The role of the antisocial family in school completion and delinquency: A three-generation study. Sociol. Quart. 7, *4*:500–514 (1966).

Robins, L.N., Murphy, G.I.: Drug use in a normal population of young Negro men. Amer. J. publ. Health 57, 1580–1596 (1967).

Robins, L.N., O'Neal, P.: The marital history of former problem children. Social Problems *5*:347–358 (1958a).

Robins, L.N., O'Neal, P.: Mortality, mobility and crime: Problem children thirty years later. Amer. Sociol. Rev. *23*:162–171 (1958b).

Robins, L.N., Wish, L.: Childhood deviance as a developmental process: A study of 223 urban black men from birth to 18. Social Forces *56*:448–473 (1977).

Robins, L.N., Bates, W.M., O'Neal, P.: Adult drinking patterns of former problem children. *In:* Society, Culture, and Drinking Patterns (D.J. Pittman and C.R. Snyder, Eds.). New York: Wiley 1962a.

Robins, L.N., Gyman, H., O'Neal, P.: The interaction of social class and deviant behavior. Amer. Sociol. Rev. *27*:480–492 (1962b).

Robins, L.N., Murphy, G.E., Breckenridge, M.B.: Drinking behavior of young urban Negro men. Quart. J. Stud. Alc. 29, *3*:657–684 (1968).

Robins, L.N., Murphy, G.E., Woodruff. R.A., Jr., King, L.J.: The adult psychiatric status of black school boys. Arch. gen. Psychiat. *24*:338–345 (1971).

Robins, L.N., West, P.A., Herjanic, B.: Arrest and delinquency in two generations: A study of black urban families and their children. J. Child Psychol. Psychiat. *16*:125–140 (1975).

Roff, M.: Relation between certain preservice factors and psychoneurosis during military duty. U.S. Armed Forces med. J. *11*:152–160 (1960).

Roff, M.: Juvenile delinquency and military service. *In:* Selective Service and American Society (R.W. Little, Ed.), New York: Russell Sage 1969.

Roff, M.: Some life history factors in relation to various types of adult maladjustment. *In:* Life History Research in Psychopathology (M. Roff and D.F. Ricks, Eds.). Minneapolis: University of Minnesota Press 1970.

Roff, M.: A two-factor approach to juvenile delinquency and the later histories of juvenile delinquents. *In:* Life History Research in Pathopathology, Vol. 2 (M. Roff, L.N. Robins, and M. Pollack, Eds.). Minneapolis: University of Minnesota Press 1972.

Rosenberg, M.: Test factor standardization as a method of interpretation. Social Forces *41*:53–61 (1962).

Rutter, M.: Autistic children: Infancy to adulthood, Semin. Psychiat. 2:435–450 (1970).

Rutter, M.L., Greenfeld, D., Lockyer, L.: A five to fifteen year follow-up study of infantile psychosis: II. Social and behavioural outcome. Brit. J. Psychiat. *113*:1183–1199 (1967).

Rutter, M., Tizard, J., Whitmore, K.: Education, Health, and Behaviour, London: Longman 1970.

Rutter, M.L., Yule, B., Quinton, D., Rowlands, O., Yule, W., Berger, M.: Attainment and adjustment in two geographical areas. III: Some factors accounting for area differences. Brit. J. Psychiat. *126*:520–533 (1975).

Rutter, M.L., Tizard, J., Yule, W., Graham, P., Whitmore, K.: Research report: Isle of Wight studies, 1964–1974. Psychol. Med. *6*:313–332 (1976a).

Rutter, M., Graham, P., Chadwick, O., Yule, W.: Adolescent turmoil: fact or fiction? J. Child Psychol. Psychiat. *17*:35–56 (1976b).

Schaie, K.W.: A reinterpretation of age related changes in cognitive structure and functioning. *In:* Life-span developmental psychology (L.R. Goulet and P.B. Baltes, Eds.). New York: Academic 1970.

Schulsinger, H.: A ten-year follow-up of children of schizophrenic mothers. Acta psychiat. scand. *53*:371–386 (1976).

Seglow, J., Kellmer Pringle, M.L., Wedge, P.. Growing up adopted. London: National Foundation for Educational Research in England and Wales 1972.

Stewart, L., Livson, N.: Smoking and rebelliousness: A longitudinal study from childhood to maturity. J. consult. Psychol. *30*:225–229 (1966).

Stewart, L.H.: Social and emotional adjustment during adolescence as related to the development of psychosomatic illness in adulthood. Genet. Psychol. Monogr. *65*:175–215 (1962).

Sudman, S., Bradburn, N.M.: Response effects in surveys. Chicago: Aldine 1974.

Terman, L.M., Oden, M.H.: The gifted child grows up. Stanford: Stanford University Press 1947.

Terman, L.M., Oden, M.H.: The gifted group at mid-life. Genetic Studies of Genius, Vol. 5. Stanford: Stanford University Press 1959.

Thomas, A., Chess, S.: Evolution of behavior disorders into adolescence. Amer. J. Psychiat. *133*:539–542 (1976).

Thomas, A., Chess, S., Birch, H.G.: Temperament and behavior disorders in children. New York: New York University Press 1968.

Tietze, C.: Fertility after discontinuation of intrauterine and oral contraception. Internat. J. of Fertility *13*:385–389 (1968).

Tuddenham, R.D., Read, D.: The constancy of personality ratings over two decades. Genet. Psychol. Monogr. *60*:3–29 (1959).

Wadsworth, M.E.M.: Delinquency, pulse rates and early emotional deprivation. Brit. J. Criminol. *16*:245–256 (1976).

Watt, N.F., Lubensky, A.W.: Childhood roots of schizophrenia. J. consult. clin. Psychol. *44*:363–375 (1976).

Watt, N.F., Stolorow, R.D., Lubensky, A.W., McClelland, D.C.: School adjustment and behavior of children hospitalized for schizophrenia as adults. Amer. J. Orthopsychiat. *40*:637–657 (1970).

Wilson, H.: Delinquency and child neglect. London: Allen and Unwin 1962.

Wolfgang, M.E., Figlio, R.M., Sellin, T.: Delinquency in a birth cohort. Chicago: University of Chicago Press 1972.

Assessing Children in Psychiatric Epidemiologic Studies

HELEN ORVASCHEL, PH.D.

DIANE SHOLOMSKAS, M.A.

MYRNA WEISSMAN, PH.D.

Introduction

Reliable epidemiologic data on rates of psychiatric disorders in children are nearly nonexistent. In particular, data are lacking on the incidence and prevalence of specific psychiatric disorders, rather than global impairment or symptoms independent of diagnosis that were characteristic of past research. Information on the rates of specific disorders would aid investigators in the identification of risk factors, advance our knowledge of etiology, contribute to the determination of treatment needs, and provide the groundwork for preventive strategies.

Rates of incidence and prevalence of psychiatric disorders cannot be based on treated populations alone. This source of data is subject to error, since many children with psychiatric disorders are likely to be untreated and therefore remain uncounted. In addition, considerable selective bias operates in determining which children are seen in treatment. For example: (1) Boys are referred for treatment more often than girls; (2) Acting-out behavior is referred more often than less overtly troublesome or withdrawn behavior; (3) Milder disorders are less likely to be treated than more severe disorders; (4) Socio-demographic variables and the availability of facilities are likely to influence who seeks and/or receives treatment. Generalizations based on clinical data are therefore, subject to distortions as to the sex and social class of the patient and the severity and type of disorder treated.

Methodological Issues

A major obstacle to epidemiologic studies of psychiatric disorders in children in the community has been the controversy regarding the reliable definition of a case. This problem is similar to previous difficulties encountered in epidemiologic studies of adult psychiatric disorders. However, there have been major achievements in the field of adult psychopathology which recently have been applied to community epidemiologic studies (Weissman and Klerman, 1978). These achievements include improved concepts, definitions, and criteria for adult psychiatric disorders such as the Research Diagnostic Criteria (RDC), American Psychiatric Association Diagnostic and Statistical Manual-Third Edition (DSM-III), and the Feighner Criteria (Feighner et al., 1972). Such advances in definition have accelerated research in adult psychiatric epidemiology by reducing the problem of criteria variance in diagnosis (Spitzer et al., 1978). This work in the classification of disorders has now been expanded to include psychiatric disorders of children (i.e., G.A.P. DSM-III), and will eventually have a similar impact on research in child psychiatric epidemiology.

Advances in adult psychiatry have also been made in techniques for symptomatic, behavioral, and diagnostic assessments. These structured assessment tools include the Schedule for Affective Disorders and Schizophrenia (SADS), the Present State Exam (PSE), and the Diagnostic Interview Schedule (DIS) (Spitzer and Endicott, 1978; Wing et al., 1974; Robins, 1979). Such techniques have reduced information variance in assessment and have resulted in considerable improvements in the reliability of psychiatric diagnosis (Endicott and Spitzer, 1978). In an effort to extend these procedures to psychiatric disorders of children, several useful scales have been developed to assess psychopathology in children.

Assessment Techniques

This chapter will review five instruments which use direct interview techniques and seem promising for epidemiologic studies of children. Although these scales are at varying stages of instrument development and most have not yet been tested in the community, they all reflect advances in the construction of standardized assessment tools suitable for survey research.

The many self-report scales and symptom checklist inventories available that are generally administered to parents, teachers, or other adults about the child have been excluded from this review for several reasons. Self-reports are more vulnerable to response biases by subjects and less amenable to qualitative information gathering than interview techniques. They do not allow for standardized observational evaluations by trained professionals, so that assessments of observable behaviors such as motor activity, immaturity, and abnormal speech patterns become problematic. In addition, certain areas of functioning are more difficult to assess by self-report measures. This is particularly true for psychiatric symptomatology which may appear in the context of mania, depression, schizophrenia, or some other psychiatric disorder. The limitations of self-reports may be especially severe if a measure is not designed to be completed by the child, who may be an important source of information concerning subjective experiences such as anxiety, depression, guilt, and the like (Herjanic et al., 1975). Self-reports do offer a number of advantages (i.e., cost, time) and it is not our intention to argue against their use. However, interview techniques overcome many of the limitations of self-reports, while providing the flexibility of information gathering often needed when dealing with less-established areas of investigation such as child psychiatric epidemiology.

In selecting which interview schedules to present in this review, our guiding criterion was their suitability for or adaptability to epidemiologic research. The following criteria were also included in our selection decision: (1) coverage of a broad spectrum of diagnostic categories or behavioral dimensions, rather than concentration on a circumscribed number of symptoms or disorders (interviews concerned primarily or exclusively with depression, anxiety, or hyperactivity were excluded, as were other single focus interviews); (2) inclusion of milder disorders as well as more severe forms of pathology; (3) use of items that are relatively defined and allow for quantitative analysis; (4) utilization of the child as one of the sources of information; and (5) existence of some reported reliability data; most scales are in the process of additional testing and refinement.

Three of the interviews (the Diagnostic Interview for Children and Adolescents, the Kiddie-SADS, and the Isle of Wight Inventory) are structured according to a categorical approach. These interviews are designed to ascertain the presence of symptoms associated with a specific psychiatric disorder. The remaining two instruments (the Mental Health Assessment Form and the Screening Inventory) utilize primarily a dimensional approach to assess overall symptomatology without grouping symptoms according to typology. The dimensional approach may be advantageous in that it allows the investigator to use linear multiple regression analysis for prediction. Multiple regression is a statistically powerful technique which does not employ the decision trees or *a priori* assumptions regarding typology that are applied to categorical instruments.

On the other hand, the use of multivariate statistical techniques (e.g., discriminant function analysis) will also provide predictive information and may be used with categorical data. The multivariate approach does not require that the data meet many of the assumptions necessary for linear regression (i.e., normality, linearity and additivity) and is superior in its handling of interactive effects between predictor variables (Paykel et al., 1973). A categorical orientation has the additional advantage of being conceptually similar to the framework used in psychiatry for research on etiology and treatment. Given that both approaches to assessment (categorical and dimensional) have advantages and limitations, the investigator must decide whether one or the other or some combination of the two meets the needs of the particular epidemiologic study in question.

The five interview schedules selected will be reviewed as to their primary purpose, scale properties, structure and content, prior use, and psychometric properties. A brief discussion of their limitations and present status is also provided.

Diagnostic Interview for Children and Adolescents

The Diagnostic Interview for Children and Adolescents (DICA) was developed by Herjanic and Welner. It is a structured psychiatric interview, with a categorical orientation, and is designed as a diagnostic instrument for children between the ages of 9 and 17 years. In a more preliminary version it was known as the Children's Psychiatric Interview (CPI) and was used with 6- to 16-year-old children. The current DICA is a considerable improvement over the CPI, but is still under revision and must be considered preliminary.

The DICA is administered directly to the child by an interviewer. A parallel form is available that is administered to the parent about the child. It requires approximately 1 to 1½ hours to complete and assesses psychiatric symptomatology during the child's lifetime. The interview is precoded and contains a complex scoring system. The DICA begins with basic demographic questions and inquiries about school functioning, relationships at home, and general interpersonal functioning. It covers the diagnostic categories of Conduct Disorder, Drug and Alcohol Abuse, Depression, Mania, Phobias, School Phobia, Obsessions and Compulsions, Anxiety Neurosis, Briquet's,

Depersonalization/Derealization, and Psychosis. Questions on enuresis and encopresis are included, in addition to sections dealing with sexuality, insight, judgment, orientation, and memory.

Analysis of this interview has thus far been reported only for the preliminary CPI version. The CPI was administered to 30 boys and 20 girls (aged 6 to 16 years), selected at random from a children's mental health clinic (Herjanic et al., 1975). Interrater reliability scores ranged from .80 to .95 with a mean of .89. Co-ratings showed an average agreement of .84. Comparisons of parent and child responses (for parallel instruments) showed an average agreement between items of 80%. No significant differences were found for content by age group, although, by sex, girls showed a consistently higher level of agreement with their parents. Testing to establish discriminant validity has been promising and attempts at obtaining diagnostic validity are in process (Herjanic and Campbell, 1976).

The DICA should be considered a very promising diagnostic instrument with considerable epidemiologic potential. Questions are well phrased and diagnostic categories appear theoretically sound. The authors are aware that further testing and refinement are necessary and are in the process of collecting the necessary data (Herjanic, 1979).

Mental Health Assessment Form

The Mental Health Assessment Form (MHAF) was developed by Kestenbaum and Bird (1979) as a screening instrument for the clinical assessment of school aged children (7 to 12 years old). It has a dimensional orientation to symptomatology and was originally designed as a tool for collecting standardized data on a sample of children with schizophrenic parents, in order to identify vulnerability to pathology.

The MHAF is not actually a psychiatric interview but, rather, a rating form that is used as an outline, around which a semistructured interview is conducted. The length of the interview may vary considerably although it is suggested that approximately 45 minutes are adequate. There are about 180 defined items to be rated on a variable scale with most items scored from 1 to 5 (ranging from no deviation to marked deviation). Specific instruction regarding the time period assessed is left unclear, but the items appear to refer to "current" functioning. The form is precoded and contains a separate score sheet.

The MHAF contains two major sections which are further subdivided into a number of areas. The first section is rated on the basis of the interviewer's observations of the child and includes items in the areas of physical characteristics, motoric behavior and speech, interpersonal relatedness, affect, and language and thinking. The second section of the form is rated on the basis of material the interviewer has elicited from the child during their interactions, and includes categories dealing with feeling states, interpersonal relations, dreams and fantasies, self-concept, moral judgment, and general level of adaptation.

A trained mental health professional, skilled in child interviewing techniques, is assumed to be required to do the interview and ratings. The ratings are based on "accepted clinical impressions about normality." A half-hour videotape demonstrating the use of the MHAF is available. A form for use with adolescents (ages 13 to 19) is also being developed by the authors (Bird, 1979). It contains additional items in such areas as drug abuse, alcoholism, and sexual behavior. This form is still in the preliminary phase of development.

Results of the MHAF have been reported for 35 children in the following three groups: 7 children with a schizophrenic parent; 2 children with a manic-depressive parent; and 26 children with a "normal" parent (Kestenbaum and Bird, 1978). Interviews were videotaped and independently rated by three child psychiatrists. Reliabilities among raters ranged from .43 to .94 for items on which some variance was present. High reliability was reported for items in the Feeling States, Interpersonal Relationships, Self-Concept, and Moral Judgment sections. Poor reliability was found for General Level of Adaptation and Use of Defense Mechanisms.

The items of depression, anger, anxiety, disturbed relationships with mother, aggressive behavior, covert aggression, bizarreness of dreams, and discrepancy between perceived and ideal self were found to discriminate between the children with psychiatrically disturbed parents and the children with normal parents. A validity study comparing the interview results of 30 clinic children to clinician ratings has also been completed. Preliminary findings suggest some validity on 35 items, particularly anxiety and depression. Many of the items could not be assessed because of a lack of variance in the ratings (Kestenbaum and Bird, 1979).

The MHAF requires a good deal more testing. Many of the items are unclear in meaning and have questionable placement in the text of the interview (i.e., masturbatory activity is rated as a motor behavior along with items such as tics and tremors). The ratings of many items require highly subjective interpretations of behavior by the interviewer (i.e., egocentricity, character of fantasy). These ratings could be improved if confined to the evaluation of specified and observable behaviors. Reliability scores reported thus far on the MHAF have been poor on many items. In addition, a better test of reliability for the interview as a whole would be generated by a test-retest situation, using different interviewers. Discriminant validity has yet to be demonstrated, since initial data were reported for a very small sample of children. The authors have indicated that the MHAF is still in revision and that they are attempting to improve the specificity of their scoring system.

Screening Inventory

The Screening Inventory (SI) was developed by Langner, Gersten, and Eisenberg to assess psychiatric impairment in children from 6 to 18 years of age. It is designed for use in community samples as a general screening instrument rather than as a diagnostic tool. The scale has a dimensional orientation and was intended to be descriptive and to represent a wide range of behaviors with predictive value for psychiatric impairment (Greene et al., 1973).

The SI is composed of three sections: (1) the background section consisting of 11 demographic items; (2) the child section consisting of 40 child behavior items; and (3) the parental section consisting of 32 parental behavior items. There are also two forms of the SI, an M-form designed to be administered to the child's parent, and a C-form designed to be administered to the child. Direct administration of the C-form, however, is limited to children 14 years of age or older. The inventory items are specific, defined, and have precoded corresponding ratings. While the time period assessed is not clearly stated, the instrument is intended to correlate with "current impairment." The questionnaire is generally administered as a structured interview (but probably can be adapted for use as a self-report). Completion time is approximately 20 minutes for a trained interviewer. The SI is accompanied by instructions and scoring sheets, age- and sex-specific forms, and a scoring procedure.

The original SI consisted of 654 items measuring the child's functioning with parents, siblings, peers, and in school. The mothers of 1,034 randomly-selected children and 1,000 welfare-supported children were interviewed for 2 to 3 hours each. Male and female children were included in the sample which represented all age groups between 6 and 18 years. The mother's responses to the questionnaire were then evaluated by two psychiatrists who rated the child's level of impairment on a 5-point scale. Interrater reliability for total impairment was .84 (Langner et al., 1976). Of the 2,034 children in the total sample, 357 were randomly selected for an individual psychiatric interview lasting approximately 1½ hours. Psychiatrists rated these children on the same 5-point psychiatric impairment scale. Ratings based on the child's interview correlated from .33 to .48 with ratings based on the mother's interview.

The questionnaire was reduced from its original 654 items to 287 items by eliminating items with low frequencies and condensing or combining other items into composites. A principal component factor analysis with orthogonal varimax rotation was performed on the remaining items. Eventually, 7 factors were identified which correlated .73 with the total impairment scores (Gersten et al., 1976). The five items with the highest loadings on each factor were selected to represent their subscale. The seven factors were: Self-Destructive Tendencies, Mentation Problems, Conflict with Parents, Regressive Anxiety, Fighting, Delinquency, and Isolation. The multiple correlation of the subscales with overall impairment was .64. An additional five items were added to the child behavior scale bringing it to a total of 40 items, with an internal consistency of .76 and interrater reliability from .43 to .66. Five factors for the parental items are also reported: Mother Rejecting, Parental Coldness, Mother's Physical and Emotional Illness, Parents Quarreling, and Child's Mild Chronic Illness.

An additional form of the SI has recently become available. This form is known as the Family Research Project Questionnaire and is intended as a cross-cultural version of the SI C-form. It is expected to be used in a number of countries in the hopes of developing cross-national norms of child psychopathology (Katz, 1979).

The SI has a number of valuable features as a screening inventory. It contains a relatively small number of well-defined items which can be administered with adequate reliability. It also enables investigators to compare data with age- and sex-appropriate norms which have been derived from a large sample. The inventory has some limitations in that it is not intended for direct administration to children under the age of 14 and therefore relies on the parent as its primary information source. In addition, interrater reliability for the 40 child behavior items was acceptable but modest (.43 to .66) and the correlations between psychiatrist's impairment ratings for mother vs. child informants were even lower (.33 to .48).

Kiddie-SADS

The Kiddie-SADS (K-SADS) was developed by Puig-Antich and Chambers as a children's version of the Schedule for Affective Disorders and Schizophrenia developed for adults by Spitzer and

Endicott. It is a structured psychiatric interview with a categorical orientation, designed primarily as a diagnostic instrument for children between the ages of 6 and 17 years. It is administered directly to children, as well as to parents about their children, and necessitates the use of a trained interviewer. It requires approximately 45 minutes to 1½ hours to complete and assesses psychiatric symptomatology during the past month or since the onset of the illness episode in question.

The first few minutes of the K-SADS involve a semistructured interaction between the interviewer and the child, during which the nature of the problem(s) and the duration are ascertained. This discussion is followed by the structured portion of the interview, which systematically investigates the child's overall symptom picture. The K-SADS covers the following diagnostic categories: Major Depression (including subtypes), Manic Disorder, Separation Anxiety (with or without school phobia), Generalized Anxiety, Phobias, Depersonalization/Derealization, Obsessive-Compulsive Disorder, Conduct Disorder, and Schizophrenia. The coding system is defined and diagnostic decisions are based on DSM-III criteria for the particular syndrome.

Preliminary testing of the K-SADS has been reported, although the number of children involved was quite small (Puig-Antich et al., 1978). Interrater reliability was excellent for the major diagnostic syndromes and ranged from .65 to .96 for individual symptoms. Test-retests were conducted following imipramine treatment of depressed children and demonstrated that K-SADS ratings were sensitive to changes due to drug treatment. Comparisons between mother and child interviews have also been encouraging and suggest the necessity of ascertaining diagnostic information from both sources (Chambers et al., 1979).

Work on a lifetime version and an epidemiologic version of the K-SADS (K-SADS-L and K-SADS-E) are currently underway and revision of the K-SADS (current version) is also in process (Puig-Antich, 1979). Diagnostic categories are being added such as Attention Deficit Disorder, Drug and Alcohol Abuse, and Panic Disorder. Previous categories have been further refined or augmented so that diagnostic decisions may be more easily determined. Symptoms on the K-SADS-L and the K-SADS-E are rated only for their presence or absence since these versions are not concerned with treatment effects but rather with a determination of psychiatric disorders (past or present). When completed, the K-SADS-L and K-SADS-E will be useful for epidemiologic research of psychiatric disorders in children. Reliability and validity studies of the K-SADS-L and K-SADS-E are underway.

Isle of Wight Survey

The Isle of Wight Survey (IWS) was developed by Rutter and Graham in an effort to obtain systematic information about psychiatric disorders in children. Psychiatric disorder was defined by the authors as " . . . abnormalities of emotions, behaviour or relationships which are developmentally inappropriate and of sufficient duration and severity to cause persistent suffering or handicap to the child and/or distress or disturbance of the family or community . . ." (Rutter and Graham, 1968, p. 153). The instrument was intended to be of diagnostic utility and was designed to elicit information directly from children between the ages of 7 and 12 years.

The IWS is a semistructured interview of approximately a half-hour's duration which utilizes both a categorical and dimensional approach. It contains over 100 items dealing with interpersonal and behavioral aspects of the child's life. Initial questions focus on school, peer contacts, family interactions, and sparetime activities. Following this, the child is assessed on behavior more specifically related to symptomatology, such as antisocial activities, hypochondriasis, fears, worries, and depression. Items are rated on a scale which varies from yes/no to a 4- or 5-point range. The time perspective of the interview is unclear, but appears to emphasize "current" behavior. When the interview is completed the interviewer rates the child for probable, definite, or no psychiatric disorder, and also indicates the nature of the disorder, if one is present.

To examine test-retest reliability, the IWS was administered to 89 children at two points in time using different interviewers. Agreement between interviewers for the rating of definite psychiatric disorder was .84 and for probable disorder was .51. Reliability scores for individual items were much lower, however, particularly for behaviors such as mood, attention, and activity. Additional examination of test-retest reliability showed good agreement for the extremes of behavior and was less favorable on more moderate item variation. Interrater reliability was tested on 25 children between the ages of 7 and 12 years and produced item agreement which ranged from .63 to .95. Discriminant validity was examined by comparing the interview findings for a normal population of 159 children with those of a population of 108 children considered psychiatrically disturbed on the basis of information obtained from parents and teachers. Interviewers were blind to the child's psychiatric status prior to the interview. Differentiation between the groups was good with psychiatric disorder ratings occurring far more frequently in the abnormal group than in the control group.

The IWS was an important first step in the development of a

psychiatric interview for use with preadolescent children. It achieved acceptable reliability scores on overall impairment ratings and was a useful tool for the initial discrimination between children with and without a psychiatric disorder. The interview did have difficulty obtaining good interrater agreement for many items and areas of functioning. This was due probably to shortcomings in the manner in which many questions were worded and the need for a more clearly defined rating system. The IWS was not always systematic in obtaining information for a particular diagnostic entity and the criteria for arriving at a diagnostic determination were not always clearly defined.

Conclusions

The five interviews reviewed do not exhaust the assessment instruments available for use with children. They are presented as an overview of the state of the art of interview techniques suitable for psychiatric epidemiology with children. All five interviews differ in basic structure, theoretical premise, and underlying diagnostic criteria (Feighner Criteria, RDC, DSM-III, ICD-9). The Screening Inventory, The Mental Health Assessment Form and to a lesser extent the Isle of Wight Survey are designed to assess overall functioning and impairment. They may be viewed as first line screening tools and would more than likely require follow-up assessments of identified cases in order to determine rates of specific disorders. The Diagnostic Interview for Children and Adolescents and the Kiddie-SADS are designed to function as basic screening devices which at the same time assign cases to discrete diagnostic categories. All the instruments require further testing and refinement and most of this is already underway. The advantages and disadvantages of a particular instrument have been discussed previously. The selection of one instrument over another must be based on the investigator's own theoretical orientation and the needs of the study for which it is intended.

Acknowledgments

This work was supported in part by Contract ADM 42-74-83 (DBE) from the Center for Epidemiologic Studies, National Institute of Mental Health, Alcohol, Drug Abuse, and Mental Health Administration (ADAMHA), Rockville, Maryland, and USPHS Research Grant #1 R01 MH28274.

References

Bird, H.R.: Personal Communication, 1979.

Chambers, W.J., Puig-Antich, J., and Tabrizi, M.A.: The ongoing development of the Kiddie-SADS. Unpublished manuscript, 1979.

Endicott, J., and Spitzer, R.L.: A diagnostic interview: The schedule for affective disorders and schizophrenia. *Arch. Gen. Psychiat.*, *35*:837–844, 1978.

Feighner, J.P., Robins, E., Guze, S.B., Woodruff, R.A., Winokur, G., and Mumoz, R.: Diagnostic criteria for use in psychiatric research. *Arch. Gen. Psychiat.*, *26*:57–63, 1972.

Gersten, J.C., Langner, T.S., Eisenberg, J.G., Simcha-Fagan, O., and McCarthy, E.D.: Stability and change in types of behavioral disturbance of children and adolescents. *J. Abn. Child Psychol.*, *4*:111–127, 1976.

Greene, E.L., Langner, T.S., Herson, J.H., Jameson, J.D., Eisenberg, J.G., and McCarthy, E.D.: Some methods of evaluating behavioral variations in children 6 to 18. *J. Amer. Acad. Child Psychiat.*, *12*:531–553, 1973.

Herjanic, B.: Personal Communication, 1979.

Herjanic, B., and Campbell, W.: Differentiating psychiatrically disturbed children on the basis of a structured interview. Unpublished manuscript, 1976.

Herjanic, B., Herjanic, M., Brown, F., and Wheatt, T.: Are children reliable reporters? *J. Abn. Child Psychol.*, *3*:41–48, 1975.

Katz, M.: Personal Communication, 1979.

Kestenbaum, C.J., and Bird, H.R.: The Mental Health Assessment Form: An instrument for the assessment of the latency age child—interrater reliability study. Unpublished manuscript, 1979.

Kestenbaum, C.J., and Bird, H.R.: A reliability study of the mental health assessment form for school age children. *J. Amer. Acad. Child Psychiat.*, *17*:338–347, 1978.

Langner, T.S., Gersten, J.C., McCarthy, E.D., Eisenberg, J.G., Greene, E.L., Herson, J.H., and Jameson, J.D.: A screening inventory for assessing psychiatric impairment in children 6 to 18. *J. Consult. Clin. Psychol.*, *44*:286–296, 1976.

Paykel, E.S., Prusoff, B.A., Klerman, G.L., Haskell, D., and DiMascio, A.: Clinical response to amitriptyline among depressed women. *J. Nerv. Ment. Dis.*, *156*:149–165, 1973.

Puig-Antich, J., Blau, S., Marz, N., Greenhill, L.L., and Chambers, W.: Pre-pubertal major depressive disorders: A pilot study. *J. Amer. Acad. Child Psychiat.*, *17*:695–707, 1978.

Puig-Antich, J.: Personal Communication, 1979.

Robins, L.N.: Diagnostic Interview Schedule. Developed under contract from the Center for Epidemiologic Studies, National Institute of Mental Health, ADAMHA, Rockville, Maryland, 1979.

Rutter, M., and Graham, P.: The reliability and validity of the psychiatric assessment of the child. I. Interview with the child. *Brit. J. Psychiat.*, *114*:563–579, 1968.

Spitzer, R.L., and Endicott, J.: Schedule for Affective Disorders and Schizophrenia. National Institute of Mental Health, Clinical Research Branch, Collaborative Program on the Psychobiology of Depression, Third Edition, May, 1978.

Spitzer, R.L., Endicott, J., and Robins, E.: Research diagnostic criteria: Rationale and reliability. *Arch. Gen. Psychiat.*, *35*:773–782, 1978.

Weissman, M.M., and Klerman, G.L.: Epidemiology of mental disorders. *Arch. Gen. Psychiat.*, *35*:705–712, 1978.

Wing, J.K., Cooper, J.E., and Sartoruis, N.: *The Measurement and Classification of Psychiatric Symptoms*. London: Cambridge University Press, 1974.

What is Child Psychiatric Epidemiology the Epidemiology Of?

THOMAS M. ACHENBACH, PH.D.

Pretend for a moment that child psychopathology is like cancer. Many individuals and families are touched by it but react in very different ways. It takes such diverse forms that there may in fact be few links among them. Its costs to society are enormous. Therapies abound, but causes and cures are elusive. The need for knowledge of incidence, prevalence, distribution, and risk factors is obvious.

If our topic were in fact cancer, our fantasy scenario would culminate in sophisticated epidemiologic studies. These, in turn, would interface with etiological, treatment, and outcome research. In child psychopathology, however, the lack of accepted definitions for the disorders themselves has hindered the convergence of research strategies. Although a few disorders have been operationally defined for research purposes, most have not received operational definitions commanding broad consensus. The lack of accepted definitions may be due not only to the rudimentary state of our knowledge, but also to the nature of the disorders themselves. Efforts to operationally define organic diseases such as cancer raise technical problems of measurement, but the existence of the disease is rarely questioned. By contrast, the paucity of known organic correlates and the lack of consensus on the nature of child psychopathology kindle endless controversies over the very existence of the disorders.

Universally acceptable measures will not emerge without consensus on what is to be measured. Must epidemiologic research therefore wait for such a consensus? It is my aim to show that epidemiologic research is not only possible without total consensus on definitions but that it may be a needed step in formulating valid definitions.

Some Sources of Confusion

Confusion often arises from differences in levels of discourse pertaining to child psychopathology. Family therapists, for example, see children's problems as symptoms of a disordered family system; the family rather than the child is thus their main focus of treatment. Yet, to find out how many children need treatment (family or otherwise), we do not need a total picture of the family dynamics of every child in a population. Similarly, psychoanalysts may consider overt symptoms to be but surface manifestations of unconscious conflict. Yet, we need not diagnose the unconscious conflicts in order to ascertain the prevalence of overt symptoms. Behavioral, organic, developmental, pedagogical, sociological, and eclectic approaches may likewise differ in their conceptions of disorders and their treatment methods but may nevertheless benefit from epidemiologic findings on overt symptoms.

Another potential source of confusion is the tendency to extrapolate too broadly a diagnostic model that may be appropriate for some disorders but not necessarily for all. For example, a few disorders—such as infantile autism, anorexia nervosa, and obsessive-compulsive states—may be sufficiently cohesive to justify a "disease entity" conception of child psychopathology. That is, the symptom pictures, developmental contexts, and other features are sufficiently uniform and striking to suggest a unitary, diseaselike phenomenon. However, only a small portion of disturbed children manifest syndromes of this sort, and, even among those who do, mixed and borderline cases are common. It remains to be seen whether further research will increase the proportion of children who can be diagnosed in terms of focalized syndromes or whether other types of diagnostic constructs will be needed.

The problem is to forge an epidemiologic data base sufficiently objective, broad, and informative to serve therapists who differ in the kinds of children they see, the contexts in which they see them, and the theoretical lenses through which they see them. The need for reaching and assessing large representative samples of children makes it necessary to concentrate on readily available data, at least until we have diagnostic constructs commanding enough consensus to warrant more intensive approaches.

Multiaxial Perspectives

DSM-III (American Psychiatric Association, 1980) is designed to broaden psychiatric taxonomy by adding four new axes to a syndromic nosology. How these axes will be used in practice remains to be seen. However, they highlight the need to view disorders in terms of overall adaptation rather than as circumscribed aberrations. Children's dependence on adults and their varying developmental status make it especially necessary to assess their overall adaptive patterns and may necessitate diagnostic concepts different from those of adult psychopathology.

Multiaxial approaches broaden diagnosis by supplementing symptom syndromes with other aspects of functioning. Yet symptom syndromes still provide the taxonomic framework within which the supplementary axes are to be used. Most of the DSM adult syndromes are rooted in familiar nosological tradition, but the child syndromes lack such a heritage. Some may prove viable but others probably will not survive. Until we accumulate research and clinical experience with the child syndromes, we will not know how reliable they are or how well they reflect differences in etiology, prognosis, or management needs.

As experience with DSM-III grows, the need for revision of its child syndromes will no doubt become evident. Therefore it may be premature to base epidemiologic research on them. Yet epidemiologic research can help improve the DSM by showing which syndromes actually occur with significant frequency, how they are distributed, how they overlap with one another, and what correlates they have. Some syndromes that made intuitive sense to the DSM Task Force, for example, may not in fact be cohesive enough to deserve syndrome status. Conversely, the DSM may omit other identifiable syndromes. Certain specific abnormalities may also deserve recognition even if they do not covary consistently enough with other abnormalities to form a syndrome. How can epidemiologic research be most fruitful under these circumstances?

Hierarchical Perspectives

Multiaxial approaches offer one way to broaden diagnosis beyond a syndromic nosology. Without a well-validated nosology, however, the value of epidemiologic data would be enhanced if they could be analyzed at multiple levels, rather than only in terms of *a priori* syndromes. The most molecular level would be specific signs and symptoms. Data of this sort are needed for syndromal diagnosis in any event, but are also important in their own right. Furthermore, they can be scored objectively and analyzed to reveal higher order patterns. Some of these higher order patterns may correspond to syndromes already recognized in a nosology such as the DSM. Other patterns may not correspond directly to such syndromes. Yet, because they are based on actual statistical associations among more molecular data, they can serve as operational definitions of syndromes whose prevalence, distribution, and correlates can be assessed. (I use the term "syndrome" in the generic sense of items that tend to occur together.)

Findings on empirically-derived syndromes can be compared with findings generated by other taxonomic approaches such as the DSM to determine which approaches are most fruitful and how different approaches can be related to one another. The most informative and reliable levels of analysis in a hierarchy can also be determined empirically. If no one level proves optimal for all purposes, different levels may be retained for different purposes. The point is that objectively scorable molecular items can serve as a foundation for deriving higher order patterns and that hierarchical relations among levels can enhance the heuristic and practical value of epidemiologic data.

Approaches to Hierarchical Analysis—One of the most elementary ways to assess associations among molecular items is with correlation coefficients. For items scored as present-versus-absent, a correlation coefficient shows the degree to which two items occur together. For items scored quantitatively, a correlation reflects covariation between the intensities or frequencies of the items.

Correlations between individual items sometimes may be useful for testing hypothesized relationships. For example, clinical lore regarding relations between firesetting and bedwetting would predict that these two items should be correlated significantly. Correlations between items may also suggest new hypotheses or may serve as nodal points around which to organize nosological impressions. However, correlations between individual items yield data only slightly less molecular than individual signs and symptoms.

To detect higher order relationships, multivariate statistical techniques can be applied to the correlations among items. Factor analysis and cluster analysis are the most widely used approaches. (See Achenbach, 1978, for a more detailed nontechnical discussion of these methods.)

Factor Analysis of Items

There are many variants of factor analysis and its close cousin, principal components analysis. We will use the terminology of factor analysis, but substituting the word "component" for "factor" would make most of the following section equally applicable to principal components analysis.

The most common factor analytic approach begins with a matrix of correlations among specific items, test scores, and/or other variables. A computer program then uses a mathematical formula to construct factors that summarize the covariation among the items in the matrix. Each factor is a vector (or dimension) composed of quantitative weights (loadings) for each of the items in the matrix. An item's loading is like a correlation coefficient that can range from −1.00 to +1.00. The loading indicates the degree to which the item correlates with the dimension represented by the factor.

When the number of items analyzed is large, many factors may be needed to represent all the dimensions of covariation among the items. The most useful factor analyses are typically those in which each factor has a few items with high loadings and many items with low loadings. The items having high loadings are the ones whose mutual covariation is most influential in determining the factor. A group of items having high loadings on a particular factor can be regarded as a syndrome in the generic sense of entities that tend to occur together. Various quantitative transformations (known as rotations) are applied to initial factor analytic results to sharpen the syndromelike groupings of items.

Second-Order Factor Analysis— If specific items are viewed as the lowest level in a hierarchy of data, and correlations among the items are a slightly higher level reflecting relations between pairs of items, then factors are a still higher level reflecting groups of intercorrelated items. The hierarchy can be extended still higher by performing second-order factor analysis of the first-order factors already obtained. This is done by computing factor scores for each individual in a sample. A factor score is a composite score based on the relations among items revealed by a particular factor. To compute the most orthodox type of factor score, an individual's raw score on each item is multiplied by the loading it received on the factor in question. These weighted raw scores are then summed; this sum is the individual's factor score for that factor.

Note that the factor score is a composite score composed of an individual's scores on all items weighted according to their loadings on a factor. This weighted combination thus reflects the dimension defined by the factor. A factor score can be computed for each factor obtained in an analysis. If seven factors are obtained in an analysis of 100 variables, for example, seven factor scores can be computed for each subject having data on the 100 variables. Each factor score is a different weighted combination of the 100 variables, and each reflects a different dimension of the data. If the factors are interpreted as reflecting schizophrenia, antisocial personality, depression, hysteria, paranoia, mania, and brain damage, for example, factor scores indicate how strongly an individual manifests each disorder.

There is also an easier way to translate factors into scores for individuals: items with high loadings on a factor are used as a scale to represent the syndrome reflected by that factor. First, a lower limit—such as .30—is chosen for the loadings to be accepted as indicating substantial covariation with the syndrome. All the items exceeding this limit on a factor are then used to define the syndrome, without differential weighting. Using just the items with loadings $\geqslant .30$, a quasi-factor score is computed by summing an individual's scores on these items.

Beside being much simpler than computing factor scores by differentially weighting every item, quasi-factor scores have two statistical advantages. One is that applying equal (unitary) weights to all items with substantial loadings preserves the most reliable distinction among loadings—the distinction between items with high loadings and those with low loadings. This may be preferable to weighting every item by its actual loading because the precise values of loadings are often unreliable (Wainer, 1976). The second advantage of quasi-factor scores is that they comprise only the items that really define each factor. By contrast, when a factor has many items with low loadings and they are all used to compute the factor score, the items with low loadings affect the factor score even though they are but marginally associated with the syndrome defining that factor.

Whichever way factor scores are computed, they can be intercorrelated, and the intercorrelations among them can be factor analyzed to produce second-order factors. Whereas a first-order factor consists of loadings for intercorrelated items, a second-order factor consists of loadings for the first-order factors whose factor scores were analyzed. Second-order factors reveal groupings of interrelated first-order factors just as first-order factors reveal groupings of interrelated items. If factors are viewed generically as syndromes, then first-order factors can be regarded as narrow band syndromes, while second-order factors are broader band syndromes comprised of interrelated narrow band syndromes.

As an example of a data hierarchy ranging from molecular items to second-order factors, consider fig. 1. The figure is based on our findings with the Child Behavior Checklist, which contains 20 social competence items and 118 behavior problem items designed to be reported by parents of children aged 4 through 16 (Achenbach, 1979). In order to reflect differences in the patterning and prevalence of problems for children of each sex at different ages, we have factor analyzed the behavior problems reported for clinically referred children of each sex in the age ranges 4–5, 6–11, and 12–16. Figure 1 depicts relations between specific behavior problems, first-order

FIGURE 1

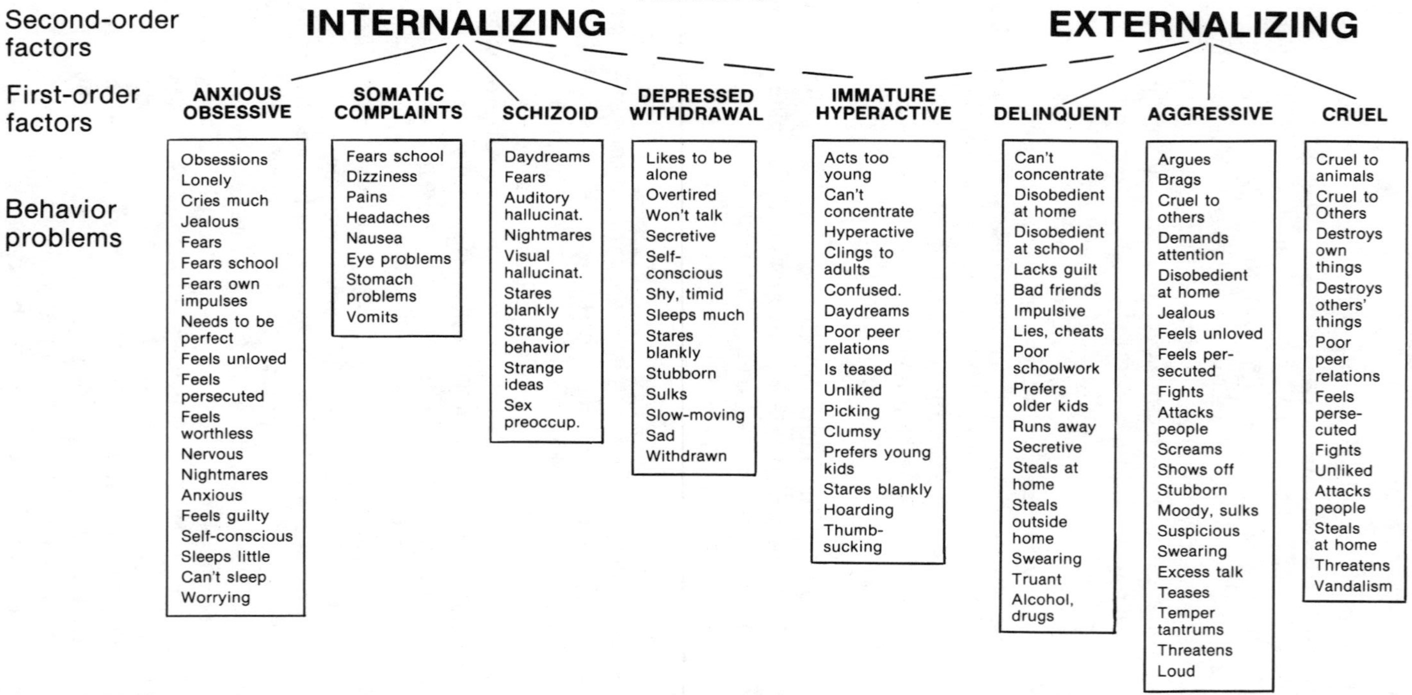

Relations between specific behavior problems, first-order factors, and second-order factors derived from the Child Behavior Checklist for girls aged 12–16.

factors, and second-order factors obtained for girls aged 12–16 (Achenbach and Edelbrock, 1979). Although 118 behavior problems were scored, not all of them were frequent enough or covaried consistently enough with other items to attain substantial loadings on a first-order factor. The items shown in fig. 1 are the ones that had loadings ⩾.30 on the first-order factor under which they are listed. Those few items that had loadings ⩾.30 on more than one factor are listed under each such factor. The factor names are intended as descriptive summaries of the problems they subsume. Some resemble traditional diagnostic categories, but others do not. The factor we labeled Cruel, for example, has no clear counterpart in traditional nosology. Its presence among girls also contradicts sex role stereotypes. Yet we found a similar factor for 6–11-year-old girls and no such factor for boys of any age.

In our second-order factor analysis, the first-order Anxious Obsessive, Somatic Complaints, Schizoid, and Depressed Withdrawal factors were found to group together with high loadings on a second-order factor we call Internalizing. By contrast, the first-order Delinquent, Aggressive, and Cruel factors grouped together with high loadings on another second-order factor that we call Externalizing. The remaining first-order factor—Immature Hyperactive—was not so exclusively aligned with either second-order factor, but had moderate loadings on both.

The Internalizing–Externalizing dichotomy clearly corresponds to a longstanding distinction among global behavior patterns in disturbed children. Although receiving different names, such as "acting out vs. overinhibited" and "personality problems vs. conduct problems," a similar dichotomy has been found in numerous empirical studies of interrelations among child behavior problems. (See Achenbach and Edelbrock, 1978, for a review of such studies.)

Obtaining epidemiologic data on relatively objective molecular items and assessing their covariation through multivariate methods such as factor analysis permits using the data at several levels. In the example shown in fig. 1, the second-order factors correspond to a coarse but widely used distinction among children's behavior problem patterns, whereas the first-order factors correspond roughly to a syndromal taxonomy like that of DSM-III. A syndrome-by-syndrome comparison of DSM-III with empirically derived first-order syndromes for children has shown moderate overlap, but there are some omissions of empirically identified syndromes from the DSM and the inclusion of some syndromes in the DSM that have not been detected by multivariate methods (Achenbach, 1980). Further research on the correlates of the DSM and empirically derived syndromes is needed to determine which ones are the most fruitful for particular purposes.

An advantage of the empirically derived syndromes for large scale epidemiologic studies is that they can be quickly and objectively scored simply by summing the scores of items defining a syndrome, as outlined above for quasi-factor scores. This can also be done for the broad band second-order syndromes by summing the items of the first-order syndromes that comprise a second-order syndrome. We have followed this strategy in computing prevalence rates on samples of 1300 normal children and 1300 disturbed children at the level of specific items, first-order factors, and second-order factors (Achenbach, 1979; Achenbach and Edelbrock, 1980). We have also computed the variance in these scores that is accounted for by age, sex, race, SES, and clinical status.

To provide a more comprehensive picture of each child's behavior pattern, we have organized our empirically derived behavior problem syndromes (and social competence scales) in a profile format called the Child Behavior Profile (Achenbach, 1979). Separate editions of the profile have been standardized for each sex at ages 4–5, 6–11, and 12–16. Because overall profile patterns may yield information not obtainable from the analysis of item and syndrome scores, the profiles themselves can be used in a taxonomic fashion for purposes of epidemiology, other types of research, and clinical evaluation, as discussed next.

Cluster Analysis of Profiles

Whereas factor analysis of items produces dimensions on which each item obtains a loading, other multivariate approaches can be used to form groupings of individuals. We have done this by cluster analyzing Child Behavior Profiles scored for large samples of disturbed children. Although there are many variants of cluster analysis, centroid linkage has been especially effective with behavioral data scored on multiple dimensions like those of the Child Behavior Profile (see Edelbrock, 1979).

In applying the centroid linkage algorithm, the clustering program first seeks the two members of a sample whose profiles are most similar to one another. Various criteria for similarity can be used, but we have found the Pearson product–moment correlation and the one-way intraclass correlation to be the best with profile data. When used as a measure of similarity between the profiles of Subject A and Subject B, a correlation is computed by treating Subject A's scores on the scales of the profile as if they were a set of observations on a single variable. Subject B's scores on the profile are treated as if they were a set of scores on a second variable.

As an example, the behavior problem portion of the Child Behavior Profile for 12–16-year-old girls comprises eight scales consisting of the items shown for the first-order factors in fig. 1. Each item is scored 0, 1, or 2 according to whether it is "not true" "somewhat or sometimes true," or "very true or often true" of the girl. The girl's scores on the items of a scale are summed to yield her raw score for that scale. The raw score is then transformed into a standard score in order to give all the scales similar means and standard deviations.

To cluster analyze profiles for a large sample of girls, correlations are computed between the eight scale scores of each girl's profile and the eight scale scores of every other girl's profile. The pair of girls whose profiles correlate highest with one another become the first cluster. The computer then sums the two girls' scores on each scale and computes the mean of each pair of scores. The result is a new eight-scale profile that is midway between the profiles of the two girls. This composite profile is called the centroid of the cluster.

After the first cluster of two cases has been formed, the program determines whether any remaining girl's profile is more similar to the cluster's centroid than to the profile of any other girl. If such a girl is found, she is added to the cluster; the cluster's centroid is then recomputed as an average of the three girls who are now members. If no unclustered girl is more similar to the centroid than to some other girl, a new cluster is started, consisting of the two most similar unclustered girls remaining in the sample. The process continues until all members of the sample are clustered or until a preset criterion is reached for clustering adequacy.

Clusters already formed can be joined to other clusters on the basis of similarity between their centroids, just as individual cases can be joined to each other and to clusters. Because the clusters are formed in a hierarchical sequence—beginning with a two-member cluster and proceeding to progressively more inclusive clusters—the hierarchy can be assessed to find the most useful levels for particular purposes. Just as with the factor analysis of items, relatively fine-grained, molecular clusters may be useful for some purposes; broader clusters subsuming molecular clusters may be useful for other purposes. Figure 2 depicts three levels in the hierarchy of clusters we found for Child Behavior Profiles of girls aged 12–16 (Edelbrock and Achenbach, 1980). The clusters at the lower levels are named in terms of the Profile scores having the highest peaks on the centroids of the clusters. Two of the clusters at the top of the hierarchy are called Internalizing and Externalizing because their

FIGURE 2

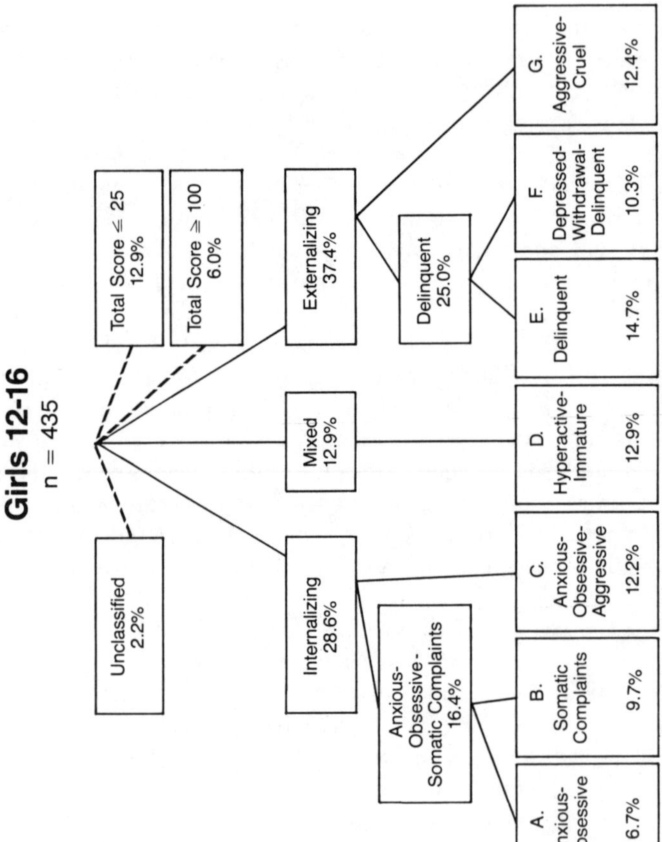

Example of a hierarchy of child behavior profile patterns found through cluster analysis.

centroids are characterized by peaks on several Internalizing or Externalizing scales respectively. The third global cluster is called Mixed because, like the Hyperactive–Immature Scale on which it has its highest peak, it is not predominantly Internalizing or Externalizing.

Although the hierarchy of factors in fig. 1 in some respects parallels the hierarchy of clusters in fig. 2, note that the latter is a hierarchy of types of profile patterns: fig. 1 reveals covariation among specific items at narrow and broad band levels of analysis, whereas fig. 2 reveals relations among groupings of narrower and broader groups of individuals. Figure 2 also shows the percentage of girls in a clinical sample (N = 435) who were classified by each profile type and the percentage left unclassified because their profile patterns were idiosyncratic or their overall scores were too low or high for meaningful classification. Such cases can be included in the typology but at the expense of reduced homogeneity within clusters. The reliability of the typology has been verified by replicating the cluster analysis in two samples of clinically referred girls and computing the correlations between the centroids of clusters obtained in the original and new samples. Only those clusters whose centroids clearly replicated are shown in fig. 2.

Because a cluster's centroid is the operational definition of the cluster, a girl not included in the original cluster analysis can be categorized by computing the correlation between her profile and the centroid of each cluster. She is then assigned to the cluster type with which her profile correlates highest. This provides an objective and reliable method for categorizing individuals according to their overall behavior problem patterns. The degree of each case's resemblance to the profile types is also indicated by the size of its correlation with the centroids of these types. This makes it possible to vary the criteria for assignment to a type according to whether broad coverage of cases is sought or whether highly homogeneous groupings are preferred at the expense of allowing more cases to remain unclassified. (See Edelbrock and Achenbach, 1980, for a detailed presentation of these issues.)

Like any other approach to taxonomy, the ultimate value of broad vs. narrow typological levels and lenient vs. stringent criteria for classification must be tested against criteria external to the taxonomy itself. We have done this by assessing relations of Child Behavior Profile types to social competence scores, demographic variables, and outcomes of mental health services (Edelbrock and Achenbach, 1980). However, studies of differential etiological factors and responsiveness to different interventions for children differing in profile type would be especially welcome tests of this (and any other) taxonomy.

Reliability of Empirically Based Taxonomies

Nosologies of the DSM type have been criticized for being unreliable. Studies of DSM adult diagnoses have shown moderate agreement for broad band categories such as neurosis versus psychosis, but declining agreement with increasing specificity of diagnosis (Sandifer et al., 1964; Tarter et al., 1975). The research-based DSM-III diagnostic criteria for adult disorders may improve reliability, but the DSM-III child nosology lacks an equivalent research base. Draft versions of the DSM-III child diagnoses have in fact shown poorer reliability than DSM-II child diagnoses (Mattison et al., 1979; Mezzich and Mezzich, 1979).

Low reliability also afflicts the Group for the Advancement of Psychiatry's (1966) system, which is tailored to children, stresses developmental factors, and is much more detailed than the DSM child nosology. Two studies of this system have shown moderate reliability only for broad band diagnoses, such as psychotic disorders, and sharp declines in reliability as specificity increased (Beitchman et al., 1978; Freeman, 1971). Agreement averaging 67% was achieved by British child psychiatrists using both the International Classification of Diseases and the Multi-axial classification drafted by the World Health Organization, but only the major broad band syndromes of these systems were employed (Rutter et al., 1975).

Important as reliability may be for other clinical and research purposes, it is especially necessary for epidemiologic studies: unless confidence can be placed in the basic data and unless these data can be combined reliably into higher order patterns, they may not be worth getting. In ordinary psychiatric diagnosis, both the lack of objective procedures for collecting basic data and for synthesizing them into a diagnostic judgment may reduce reliability. The studies of the reliability of child psychiatric diagnosis have skirted the first source of unreliability by giving all the judges exactly the same case history materials (Beitchman et al., 1978; Freeman, 1971; Mattison et al., 1979; Mezzich and Mezzich, 1979; Rutter et al., 1975). The lack of diagnostic agreement thus reflects only the differences among diagnosticians' responses to exactly the same data; had they independently obtained their own data—as is typical of actual practice—diagnostic agreement may have been lower yet.

Beside disagreements due to stable individual differences between diagnosticians, inconsistencies "within" diagnosticians may also reduce reliability. In having the same psychiatrists rediagnose the same case histories after a three-month interval, Freeman (1971) found only 72% agreement between the psychiatrists' first and second diagnoses.

Reliability of Items

Although empirically derived syndromes and profile types should be considered more as aids to diagnosis than as substitutes for it, the question of reliability is equally relevant to these approaches. We have assessed several forms of reliability for our Child Behavior Checklist and the syndromes and profile types derived from it. At the most molecular level, we obtained the following intraclass correlations (ICC) between item scores (Achenbach and Edelbrock, 1980): (a) for test–retest reliability of 72 mothers' ratings obtained by an interviewer visiting their homes at a one-week interval, ICC = .952 for behavior problems and .996 for social competence; (b) for interparent agreement between ratings by mothers and fathers of 168 children at intake into mental health settings, ICC = .985 for behavior problems and .978 for social competence; (c) for interinterviewer reliability, computed by comparing parent ratings of 241 triads of demographically matched children when the parent of each child in each triad was interviewed by a different interviewer, ICC = .959 for behavior problems and .927 for social competence; (d) for 3-month stability, assessed by having 12 mothers rerate their normal children, ICC = .838 for behavior problems and .974 for social competence. These figures indicate satisfactory reliability for the basic data on which our empirically derived syndromes and profiles rest.

Reliability of Syndromes

Scoring a child's Checklist for each syndrome type is an objective, essentially clerical, procedure. Even though deriving syndrome scores from the molecular data should be completely reliable, however, these scores are sums of various combinations of individual items. It is therefore important to assess their reliability as units. We have done this by computing Pearson product–moment correlations between total scores on the scales derived from the Checklist (Achenbach, 1979): (a) for test–retest reliability of 49 mothers' ratings obtained by a home interviewer at a one-week interval, the average correlation of the scale scores was .88; (b) for interparent agreement between mothers and fathers of 97 children at intake into mental health settings, the average correlation was .68; (c) for 6-month stability, assessed by having parents rerate 84 children seen in mental health settings, the average correlation was .72.

The Pearson correlations primarily reflect agreement in the rank ordering of scores; *t*-tests on the means of the scale scores showed negligible differences between the means obtained for mothers' ratings at one-week intervals and for the comparisons of mothers' and fathers' ratings, but general declines in behavior problem scores over 6 months for children seen for treatment. These declines—and larger declines found in 18-month follow-ups—indicate that the magnitudes of syndrome scores are sensitive to changes expected to occur with treatment.

TABLE 1

Reliability and Stability of Syndrome Ratings

		Type of Syndrome	
Type of Measure	Type of Rater	Broad Band	Narrow Band
Test-retest reliability (1 week to 1 month)	Parents	.90	.88
	Teachers	.87	.82
Short-term stability (1½ to 6 months)	Parents	.83	.77
	Teachers	.83	—
	Mental health workers	.59	.57
Long-term stability (15 months to 5 years)	Parents	.60	.52
Interrater reliability	Parents	.69	.69
	Teachers	.79	—
	Mental health workers	—	.72
Different raters seeing children in different contexts		.37	.19

Note: Figures are averages of correlations obtained in studies reported in detail by Achenbach et al., (1980) and Achenbach and Edelbrock (1978); test–retest reliabilities were not available for mental health workers' ratings nor were long-term stabilities available for mental health workers' or teachers' ratings of either broad band or narrow band syndromes.

To provide a summary overview of reliability for empirically derived syndromes, table 1 shows the average of correlations between scores for various raters on various empirically derived broad and narrow band syndromes. The component studies are described in more detail elsewhere (Achenbach et al., 1980; Achenbach and Edelbrock, 1978). Note the weakness of the correlations between different types of raters seeing children in different contexts as compared to the other correlations. This suggests that syndromal assessment is highly dependent on the context in which the child is seen and on the rater's role in relation to the child.

Reliability of Profile Types

In addition to the reliability of syndrome scores, it is also important to consider agreement between classifications according to profile types when the molecular data come from different raters. The procedure for classifying an individual Checklist according to profile types is objective, but differences between raters could produce different profile patterns for the same child. Because mothers and clinicians are usually the key informants regarding children's psychopathology, we compared the classification of profiles scored from Checklists filled out by mothers of 67 child psychiatric outpatients and Checklists filled out by a clinician who evaluated all the children (Edelbrock and Achenbach, 1980). In addition to interviews with the children and their families, the clinician had access to Checklists filled out by the mothers and in most cases the fathers, teachers, and children themselves. Although the clinician's ratings were not totally independent of the mothers' ratings, the aim was to provide the clinician with as much information as possible about the child as perceived from diverse perspectives. The clinician was to serve as a disinterested but knowledgeable outsider who would try to glean as complete and objective a picture as possible. The clinician did not know, however, what profile patterns would emerge from either the mothers' Checklist ratings or her own.

At the level of specific profile types, classification based on the mothers' Checklists agreed with those based on the clinician's Checklists for 70% of 6–11- and 12–16-year-old boys, 75% of 6–11-year-old girls, and 80% of 12–16-year-old girls. At the level of the Internalizing, Externalizing, and Mixed patterns, agreement was 95% for 6–11-year-old boys, 74% for 12–16-year-old boys, 75% for 6–11-year-old girls, and 90% for 12–16-year-old girls. Because these percentages are affected by the distribution of judgments among categories, the statistic kappa (Cohen, 1960) was computed to control for chance agreements. Ratios of the obtained kappas to the maximum kappas possible for the actual distributions among categories were 1.00 for all four age/sex groups at the Internalizing-Mixed-Externalizing level and for two of the four groups at the level of specific profile type. The remaining kappa/kappa max ratios were .811 and .897. Like traditional nosologies, agreement for broad band categories of profile patterns is thus better than for narrow band patterns, but, at both levels, agreement between mothers and a clinician were considerably higher than between clinicians for traditional nosological categories.

Validity of Empirically Based Taxonomies

The validity of a taxonomy must be judged in relation to the needs of its users. Any phenomena can be categorized in diverse ways. Where specific etiologies are known, they may provide a good basis for taxonomy, although management needs, prognosis, severity, or handicaps may be equally important taxonomic criteria. Where specific etiologies and effective treatments are not known—as in child psychopathology—taxonomies may be judged in terms of their ability to facilitate communication about individual cases and the grouping of cases for purposes of training, research, and planning. Unless a taxonomy is reliable, it cannot fulfill either the communication or the grouping function.

Beside the need for reliability, however, a taxonomy's value depends on its breadth and ease of application and on its ability to discriminate among cases differing on variables other than the taxonomy's own criterial attributes. Although the professional vocabulary embodied in nosologies of the DSM type may imply an ease of use and a face validity of sorts, there is little evidence that they in fact aid in discriminating among children who also differ consistently in other important respects. Communications about individual children typically focus more on histories, descriptions, and inferences than on firm nosological distinctions. Furthermore, communications about individual children are shaped by the professional and theoretical predilections of the clinician, as well as the context in which the children are seen.

Empirically derived taxonomies, by contrast, use data that can be readily obtained in a uniform manner across settings without much professional involvement. There is also considerable evidence that these data discriminate among children who differ in other important ways. At the most fundamental level of discrimination, scores on specific behavior problems, narrow band, and broad band syndromes have all been found significantly higher for clinically referred children than for demographically similar normal children (Achenbach, 1979; Achenbach and Edelbrock, 1980).

As for discrimination among disturbed children, it has been found that those categorized at the broad band level as Externalizers differ in the following ways from those categorized as Internalizers: Externalizers have poorer academic and standardized test performance; are rated less favorably by teachers and peers; have more premorbid social problems; display less self-control on measures of impulsivity, delay of gratification, and foresight; show less disparity between their real-self and ideal-self images; and terminate sooner and improve less in psychotherapy (Achenbach, 1966; Achenbach and Lewis, 1971; Katz et al., 1975; Rolf, 1972; Rolf and Garmezy, 1974; Weintraub, 1973).

In a long-term follow-up of disturbed adolescents in adulthood (at a mean age of 38), those initially classified as Externalizers differed from demographically matched Internalizers in the following ways (Hafner et al., 1975): Externalizers had worse academic records, completed fewer grades, were less likely to finish high school, had fewer friends, and received poorer mental health ratings. Within-sex comparisons showed less adequacy for Externalizers on indices of occupational, marital, and social adjustment. Other versions of the Internalizing-Externalizing dichotomy have also shown worse outcomes for Externalizers than Internalizers (Lorion and Cowen, 1976; Lorion et al., 1974). Furthermore, parents of Externalizers have been found to differ from parents of Internalizers in being less strict with their child and less concerned about the child's problems, and in having more overt social problems, more marital separations, more overall pathology, and different MMPI profiles (Achenbach, 1966; Achenbach and Lewis, 1971; Anderson, 1969; Weintraub, 1973).

Although research on the more differentiated patterns is in an early stage, it has found patterns related to differences in race, age, SES, school performance, and participation in activities and social relationships (Edelbrock and Achenbach, 1980). We are currently analyzing relations between profile patterns and various measures of behavioral change in children treated in outpatient and residential settings. We are also comparing profile patterns obtained from Checklist ratings by parents and ratings on companion instruments by teachers, clinicians, and trained observers to determine which ones are the best predictors of outcome.

Another approach to validating profile patterns is to compare the patterns of children receiving different clinical diagnoses. If the empirical measures and clinical diagnoses correlate well, they may be usable in tandem to provide a better basis for taxonomy than either would alone. However, failure of the empirical measures to correlate well with clinical diagnoses should not automatically lead to rejection of one approach. Instead, choices between them should be made on the basis of their reliability and their power to discriminate among children who are shown to differ on other important variables.

Conclusions

What is child psychiatric epidemiology the epidemiology of? We don't really know yet, but epidemiologic studies using a broad enough approach to data collection and analysis may help us find out. In the absence of a well-validated clinical nosology, it seems preferable to target epidemiologic research on specific signs and symptoms that (a) can be ascertained by similar methods in general population and clinical samples; (b) can be objectively scored and quantified; (c) can be analyzed in terms of multiple dimensions and hierarchical levels instead of being restricted to yes-no diagnoses; and (d) can be interfaced with other research strategies in a convergent fashion.

If the DSM-III categories of childhood disorders are scorable from data obtainable in epidemiologic surveys, then the most productive strategy may be to score both the DSM disorders and empirically derived syndromes and profiles like those illustrated in figs. 1 and 2. Relations between the two approaches then can be assessed and their distributions and correlates can be compared. High agreement between them would suggest that they could be used interchangeably or in tandem; low agreement would indicate a need for choices between them; the obtained distributions and correlates could reveal strengths or weaknesses peculiar to each approach that might aid in choosing between them. If the two approaches agreed well in some areas but not others, this could highlight particular trouble spots needing further effort.

References

Achenbach, T. M. The classification of children's psychiatric symptoms: a factor-analytic study. *Psychological Monographs* 80, 1966 (Whole No. 615).

Achenbach, T. M. *Research in developmental psychology: Concepts, strategies, methods.* New York: Free Press, 1978.

Achenbach, T. M. The Child Behavior Profile: an empirically based system for assessing children's behavioral problems and competencies. *International Journal of Mental Health*, 1979, 7:24–42.

Achenbach, T. M. DSM-III in light of empirical research on the classification of child psychopathology. *Journal of the American Academy of Child Psychiatry*, 1980, in press.

Achenbach, T. M., Dickerson, F. B., and Edelbrock, C. S. Relations between parent, teacher, and clinician reports of behavior problems in child and adolescent outpatients at intake and follow-up. Manuscript in preparation, 1980.

Achenbach, T. M., and Edelbrock, C. S. The classification of child psychopathology: A review and analysis of empirical efforts. *Psychological Bulletin*, 1978, *85*:1275–1301.

Achenbach, T. M., and Edelbrock, C. S. The Child Behavior Profile: II. Boys aged 12–16 and girls aged 6–11 and 12–16. *Journal of Consulting and Clinical Psychology*, 1979, *47*:223–233.

Achenbach, T. M., and Edelbrock, C. S. Behavioral problems and competencies reported by parents of normal and disturbed children aged 4 through 16. *Monographs of the Society for Research in Child Development*, 1980, in press.

Achenbach, T. M. and Lewis, M. A proposed model for clinical research and its application to encopresis and enuresis. *Journal of the American Academy of Child Psychiatry*, 1971, *10*:535–554.

American Psychiatric Association, Task Force on Nomenclature and Statistics. *Diagnostic and Statistical Manual of Mental Disorders.* (3rd edition). Washington, D.C.: Author, 1980.

Anderson, L. M. Personality characteristics of parents of neurotic, aggressive, and normal preadolescent boys. *Journal of Consulting and Clinical Psychology*, 1969, *33*:575–581.

Beitchman, J. H., Dielman, T. E., Landis, J. R., Benson, R. M., and Kemp, P. L. Reliability of the Group for the Advancement of Psychiatry diagnostic categories in child psychiatry. *Archives of General Psychiatry*, 1978, *35*:1461–1466.

Cohen, J. A coefficient of agreement for nominal scales. *Educational and Psychological Measurement*, 1960, *20*:37–46.

Edelbrock, C. S. Mixture model tests of hierarchical clustering algorithms: The problem of classifying everybody. *Multivariate Behavioral Research*, 1979, *14*:367–384.

Edelbrock, C. S., and Achenbach, T. M. A typology of child behavior profile patterns: Distribution and correlates for disturbed children aged 6–16. *Journal of Abnormal Child Psychology*, 1980, *8*, in press.

Freeman, M. A reliability study of psychiatric diagnosis in childhood and adolescence. *Journal of Child Psychology and Psychiatry*, 1971, *12*:43–54.

Group for the Advancement of Psychiatry. Psychopathological disorders in childhood: Theoretical considerations and a proposed classification. *Report No. 62*, 1966.

Hafner, A. J., Quast, W., and Shea, M. J. The adult adjustment of one thousand psychiatric and pediatric patients: Initial findings from a twenty-five year follow-up. In R. D. Wirt, G. Winokur, and M. Roff (Eds), *Life History Research in Psychopathology*, Vol. 4. Minneapolis: Univ. of Minnesota Press, 1975.

Katz, P. A., Zigler, E., and Zalk, S. R. Children's self-image disparity: The effects of age, maladjustment, and action-thought orientation. *Developmental Psychology*, 1975, *11*:546–550.

Lorion, R. P., Cowen, E. L., and Caldwell, R. A. Problem types of children referred to a school-based mental health program. *Journal of Consulting and Clinical Psychology*, 1974, *42*:491–496.

Lorion, R. P., and Cowen, E. L. Comparison of two outcome groups in a school-based mental health project. *American Journal of Community Psychology*, 1976, *4*:65–73.

Mattison, R., Cantwell, D. P., Russell, A. T., and Will, L. A comparison of DSM-II and DSM-III in the diagnosis of childhood psychiatric disorders: II. Inter-rater agreement. *Archives of General Psychiatry*, 1979, *36*:1217–1222.

Mezzich, A. C., and Mezzich, J. E. Diagnostic reliability of childhood and adolescence behavior disorders. Paper presented at the American Psychological Association, New York, N. Y., September, 1979.

Rolf, J. E., and Garmezy, N. The school performance of children vulnerable to behavior pathology. In D. F. Ricks, A. Thomas, and M. Roff (Eds), *Life History Research in Psychopathology*, Vol. 3. Minneapolis: Univ. of Minnesota Press, 1974.

Rolf, J. E. The social and academic competence of children vulnerable to schizophrenia and other behavior pathologies. *Journal of Abnormal Psychology*, 1972, *80*:225–243.

Rutter, M., Shaffer, D., and Shepherd M. *A Multiaxial Classification of Child Psychiatric Disorders: An Evaluation of a Proposal.* Geneva, Switzerland: World Health Organization, 1975.

Sandifer, M. G., Pettus, C., and Quade, D. A study of psychiatric diagnosis. *Journal of Nervous and Mental Disease*, 1964, *139*:350–356.

Tarter, R. E., Templer, D. I., and Hardy, C. Reliability of the psychiatric diagnosis. *Diseases of the Nervous System*, 1975, *36*:30–31.

Wainer, H. Estimating coefficients in linear models: It don't make no nevermind. *Psychological Bulletin,* 1976, *83*:213–217.

Weintraub, S. A. Self-control as a correlate of an internalizing-externalizing dimension. *Journal of Abnormal Child Psychology*, 1973, *1*:292–307.

Epidemiologic Studies of Children Problems of Screening

NAOMI RICHMAN, M.D.

Introduction

The essence of epidemiologic studies is to provide information relevant to populations either by surveying everyone or more usually by investigating carefully chosen samples from the total population. The size of the study sample will be determined by the expected rate of occurrence in the population of the problem under investigation, and the likely rate of attrition through inability to locate subjects, refusals, and losses over the study period because of moves, etc. In addition the sample must be sufficiently large to allow examination of associated independent variables of interest; for example, in studying delinquency rates one might wish to look at the effects of variations in schools, families, and neighborhood.

The simplest method of identification is to use agency or official records (e.g., rates of suicides or court appearances). Often it is not certain how complete such case finding is, and the characteristics of the population from which the cases come is not known. Only a small proportion of certain conditions may be notified; for example, in the United Kingdom about one-tenth of school children with psychiatric disorders attend psychiatrists. For these reasons it may be decided to identify subjects in the population directly.

The need for investigating large samples limits methods of data collection to those which are not too lengthy or do not involve highly expensive or skilled techniques. In order to use resources most effectively a two stage design may be chosen. In the first or screening stage a fairly simple method is used to gather data on the chosen samples and identify those with the condition to be investigated. In the second stage selected samples with and without the condition can then be examined in depth in order to validate the findings of the first stage and investigate in more detail variables associated with the problem under study and causal hypotheses (Rutter, 1977). As an example, we wanted to examine the prevalence of behavior difficulties in 3-year-old children, the natural history of these difficulties, and associated demographic and family factors. In order to do the study we decided to develop a screening interview to identify children in the community, since it was clear that most children with behavior difficulties would not be attenders at treatment facilities. We estimated that we would have to try to contact and interview approximately 1000 families in order to identify 100 children with behavior problems (Richman et al., 1975).

In another study we wished to examine the characteristics of an unselected sample of 1–2-year-olds with sleep problems. A postal questionnaire on the child's sleep to be completed by parents was used as the screen although we were aware that the likely return on a postal questionnaire is less than with personal contact. Out of 1200 questionnaires, approximately 60% were returned and of these 10% reported severe waking difficulties. Other studies have used screening questionnaires completed by teachers on samples of school children (Rutter, 1967; Rutter et al., 1970).

In both our preschool studies the sampling frame was a computerized register of all families with a child under five years living in a London borough, and we were able to screen a one in four random sample of practically the total population at risk (Richman and Tupling, 1974). Whatever the source of the sample, investigators must be aware of possible bias in its structure; for instance, nonresponders are known to have higher rates of psychiatric disorder (Cox et al., 1977). Characteristics of nonresponders to our sleep questionnaire may have been significantly different from responders.

Definition of a Case and Validity

The nature of screening inevitably produces rather simplified measures of the problem under study. This may seem inappropriate when dealing with emotional disturbance, and where the demarcation between "normal" and "abnormal" is never clear-cut. Although these limitations have to be accepted, the value or validity of the screening measure must be established, i.e., how well it can select subjects which meet the criteria chosen to define a case. In our preschool survey we used the number and severity of symptoms shown by the child to form the behavior screen whilst recognizing that this ignores qualitative differences important to clinicians. Our criterion of a case was based on clinical experience and defined as the presence of behavior in the child sufficiently handicapping or distressing to the child or family that it merited some form of help.

Methods of establishing the validity of a screening instrument include comparisons with information obtained in clinical interviews with child and family, with scores on other measures known to be valid, or with independent observations or reports on the child. These measures of concurrent validity may be supplemented by those of predictive validity, i.e. ability to predict future outcome such as high scorers on a preschool scale having difficulty in settling at school. However, low predictive validity does not necessarily mean that the scale is poor, since children are not always consistent in their development nor do they always behave in the same way in different situations. Children validly may score differently on the same scale at school and at home (Rutter et al., 1970; Minde and Minde, 1977).

The concurrent validity of the postal questionnaire on sleep was examined through detailed interviews with parents and by asking the parents to keep diaries of the child's sleep for two weeks. Both interview and diaries confirmed that the postal questionnaire was valid and did distinguish between good and bad sleepers.

The validity of our Behaviour Screening Interview was initially tested by its ability to distinguish between 3-year-old attenders at a special day center for children with behavioral difficulties and a group from the general population. (Richman and Graham, 1971).

Type of Questionnaire

Screening questionnaires can be divided into two main types, self-completed questionnaires which the informant fills in on his own completely independently (e.g., the sleep questionnaire), and interview questionnaires in which an interviewer using a standardized interview talks to the informant and makes a judgment of the presence or absence of a particular problem and its severity.

It would be impossible to exclude all bias from any screening measure. For instance, interviewers' attitudes may bias their ratings or affect the way they talk to certain parents. A depressed mother may overemphasize the difficulties she experiences with her child, a defensive one underplay them. A tendency to give all high scores because the child is difficult in one area (halo effect) or to respond in the same way (response set), e.g., by always giving the lowest or highest scores, are also sources of bias. It is particularly difficult to obtain objective and bias-free information on young children, since parents are often the only informants and it is obviously impossible for them to be emotionally detached. Indeed, the child's behavior cannot be completely independent of family interaction.

Thorough training and monitoring of interviews and carefully laid down criteria for rating help to eliminate interviewers' bias. Self-completed questionnaires eliminate interview bias but also the interviewer's skills, since the more open-ended questions used in semistructured interviews can improve sensitivity by obtaining a more detailed picture of behavior.

In our preschool study we decided to develop both interview and self-completed questionnaires so that we could compare the two. We thought a self-completed questionnaire would be easier and cheaper to use and might be able to provide a useful measure for researchers with limited resources, but a semistructured interview questionnaire would be more sensitive.

The Behavior Screening Interview or Questionnaire (BSQ) consists of questions on twelve areas of behavior which were found on piloting to be among the most common difficulties encountered by parents who sought help for their young children.

Each behavior is rated 0 if absent or infrequent, 1 if occasional or mild, 2 if severe or frequent. Carefully laid down criteria are given for each rating, and the interview is semistructured; that is, the interviewer has to ask the prescribed questions but is free to elaborate on these until he has sufficient information to rate a given behavior. A total score (the BSQ score) is calculated by adding up the ratings for each behavior, giving a range of 0 to 24. (Richman and Graham, 1971).

The Behavior Checklist (BCL) is a self-completed questionnaire filled in by a parent. It covers the same twelve areas of behavior as the BSQ and is scored in the same way. For each item the parent selects one of three descriptions which describe the child's current behavior; there is obviously no opportunity to clarify or elaborate their answers.

Reliability

If a child scored 5 on a measure one week and 15 the next this could be because his behavior was very variable. However, for screening purposes we are interested in fairly stable behavior; frequent variability in results would lead us to question the usefulness of the screen, as would inconsistent results with different interviewers. Variations in scores at different times could be due to a number of influences: a change in the child's behavior or in the mother's attitude toward the child or the screening procedure; variation in the ability of the interviewer to elicit information from the mother or to rate the behaviors.

The reliability or consistency of the BSQ was examined in two ways. Some mothers were interviewed twice by two different interviewers at roughly a week's interval (test-retest reliability), and the two interviewers listened to tape recordings of an interview carried out by one of them (interrater reliability). The two sets of ratings were compared in both cases. We found that the overall BSQ score was highly reliable, but that scores on individual items of the scale were more variable (Richman and Graham, 1971). Test-retest reliability of the BCL produced similar results (Richman, 1977a). Disagreements between the raters about classification, i.e., whether the total score fell above or below the cut off point of 10, were few, especially with BSQ. We concluded that the BSQ and BCL were adequately reliable instruments particularly with regard to the total score.

Sensitivity and Specificity

It is obviously essential to know the sensitivity or likelihood of error of a screening instrument; that is, how many "correct" cases it selects (sensitivity), how many it misses (false negatives), and how many wrong cases or false positives are selected (specificity). The absolute rates of disorder estimated will depend on the chosen cutoff point and whether one wishes to have a more sensitive measure (i.e., one that selects more cases) at the cost of reducing specificity and raising the number of false positives.

On initial standardization of the BSQ, any child scoring 11 or more points was considered at risk of having a behavior problem. For the preschool survey of 3-year-olds the cutoff point was lowered to 10 to increase sensitivity. A clinical assessment was used to judge whether 100 low scorers (BSQ < 10) and 100 high scorers (BSQ $\geqslant 10$) had been correctly identified by the screen (Richman et al., 1975). Using this criterion, it was estimated that there were 6% false positives and 10% false negatives in our community sample of 705 3-year-old children (table 1).

All the problems considered to be clinically marked in severity were selected by the BSQ; in other words, all the false negatives were mild cases. We concluded that the BSQ was highly specific and adequately sensitive, especially if only the most difficult problems were to be identified.

The BCL was completed independently by the parents before the screening interview and was found to be less useful than the BSQ. There were more false positives (13%) and false negatives (30%) and it identified only 82% of the marked problems (Richman, 1977a).

TABLE 1

Sensitivity and Specificity of Behavior Screening Questionnaire (BSQ)

	Clinical assessment		
BSQ score	Case	Non case	Total
⩾ 10	94	6 False +	100
< 10	60 False −	545	605
Total	154	551	705

False negatives	60/605 = 10%
False positives	6/100 = 6%
Sensitivity	94/154 = 61%
Specificity	545/551 = 99%
Misclassified False − and false +	66/705 = 9%

This relative insensitivity is probably because a checklist provides less clearly defined and consistent rating criteria than does an interview. This view is supported by another study comparing the BCL and BSQ scores of 125 children who were registering for junior kindergarten in Toronto (Minde and Minde, 1977). Overall agreement between the pairs of scores was fair. However it was found that if the BCL were given first, correlation was lower than if it were given second when there was nearly total agreement. The authors suggest that increased agreement is because interviewing might sensitize the parents to their child's behavior and make their thinking more systematic and specific when they completed the checklist.

Support for concurrent validity of the BSQ was given by independent behavioral ratings of high and low scorers in the preschool survey made during developmental testing by a psychologist. High and low scorers also differed in developmental, family, and social factors, showing that the BSQ was able to select a clinically distinct group of children with behavior problems (Richman, 1977c). These differences were still apparent at four and eight years on a number of different measures indicating that the BSQ also has predictive validity (Richman, 1977b; Richman et al., 1980).

Uses and Limitations of Screening Measures

The relative ease with which screening measures can be administered makes it particularly important that their use should be very carefully considered. Researchers need to know the reliability, sensitivity, and specificity, and the population used for standardization of any questionnaire they use. The validity of a questionnaire needs to be established for each new population with which it is used.

The limitations of a particular instrument must be recognized. For instance, as the BSQ has been standardized for use with parents on 3-year-old children living in England it may not be appropriate for children who are much younger or much older or who come from different social environments. The way in which a case is defined by the BSQ means that it will not select children with monosymptomatic problems however severe. The use of a three point scale for each behavioral item produces a relatively crude differentiation of severity and obscures qualitative differences.

The inability of a screening instrument to make qualitative distinctions means that children with the same scores are not necessarily equally disturbed, nor can it be assumed that a child who scores 20 on the BSQ is twice as difficult as one who scores 10. Although it is true that the group of children with the most severe problems as rated clinically have the highest mean scores on the BSQ, the type of questionnaire we are discussing is not an equal interval scale, and treating the scores as a continuous variable may not be justified statistically.

Given that the sensitivity and specificity of a given instrument is known, it can then be used in various ways. First it can identify subjects at risk as part of a two stage survey, in which case it may be wished to have a highly sensitive instrument as false positives can be recognized in the second stage. Second, it can be used to provide comparative information on rates of a disorder in different populations.

Both identification of subjects and estimates of prevalence will be improved if more than one informant is available. For instance, since children behave differently in school and at home, relying only on teachers' questionnaires probably would produce a rate approximating half the true prevalence (Rutter et al., 1975) and identify only half the children with problems. Using a parent screening questionnaire also improves accuracy of case finding and estimates of prevalence (Rutter et al., 1970).

Third, screening can provide an indicator of morbidity or need. As an example of such a use, scores on the BCL from a stratified random sample of preschool children living in England and Wales were used as one index (that of behavior difficulties) of day care need in the total population (Bone, 1977). Knowing the proportion of high scorers who are likely to be cases and the rate of false negatives gives a more accurate estimate of morbidity.

Screening instruments have very limited use clinically; results must be interpreted extremely cautiously and a high score seen only as an indicator of where further assessment might be helpful. It must always be remembered that a high score on a particular test should not be taken as definitely indicative of deviance or abnormality, since it could be a false positive; similarly, a low score could be a false negative. Even less weight can be attached to scores for individual behavioral items which are known to be less reliable.

Finally there are ethical problems in intruding on families who have not sought contact or asked for help. Investigators must also decide what to do when serious problems are identified. In our sleep study we actually offered help to all participants if they wished for it. In the preschool behavior study, however, we contacted sources of help only where the families requested this and where we felt the problem was extremely serious, but decisions about what to do were often extremely difficult.

References

Bone M. 1977 Preschool children and the need for day-care. HMSO London.

Cox, A., Rutter, M., Yule, B., et al. Bias resulting from missing information: some epidemiological findings. Br. J. Prev. Soc. Med. 31(2):131–6.

Minde R. and Minde K. (1977) Behavioral screening of preschool children: A new approach to mental health? in ed. P.J. Graham Epidemiological Approaches in Child Psychiatry. Academic Press, London. pp. 139–164.

Richman N. and Graham P.J. (1971) A behavioural screening questionnaire for use with three-year-old children: preliminary findings. J. Child Psychol. Psychiat. *12*:5–33.

Richman N. and Tupling H. (1974) A computerised family register of children under five in a London Borough. Health Trends *6*:19–22.

Richman N., Stevenson J.E., Graham P.J. (1975) Prevalence of behaviour problems in three-year-old children: an epidemiological study in a London borough. J. Child Psychol. Psychiat. *16*:277–287.

Richman N. (1977a) Is a behaviour checklist for preschool children useful? in ed. P.J. Graham Epidemiological Approaches in Child Psychiatry Academic Press, London. pp. 125–137.

Richman N. (1977b) Short term outcome of behaviour problems in 3 year old children. in ed. P.J. Graham Epidemiological Approaches in Child Psychiatry. Academic Press, London pp. 165–178.

Richman N. (1977c) Behaviour problems in preschool children: family and social factors. Br. J. Psychiat. *131*:523–527.

Richman N., Stevenson J.E., Graham P.J. (1980) (In preparation).

Rutter M. (1967) A children's behaviour questionnaire for completion by teachers: preliminary findings. J. Child Psychol. Psychiat. *8*:1–11.

Rutter M., Tizard J., Whitmore K. (1970) Education, Health and Behaviour. London: Longman.

Rutter M., Cox A., Tupling C., Berger M., Yule W. (1975) Attainment and adjustment in 2 geographical areas 1. The prevalence of psychiatric disorder. Br. J. Psychiat. *128*:493–509.

Rutter M. (1977) Surveys to answer questions: some methodological considerations in ed. P.J. Graham Epidemiological Approaches in Child Psychiatry. Academic Press, London. pp. 1–30.

Methodological Problems in Cross-Cultural Epidemiologic Research: Illustrations from a Survey of Childhood Autism in Africa

VICTOR LOTTER, PH.D.

Psychiatric epidemiology aims to establish prevalence rates for disorders in different populations. One of the uses of the information collected is the exploration of risk factors. Difficulties of psychiatric case definition are notorious, discouraging epidemiologic investigations, especially into disorders of childhood (Graham, 1978). In cross-cultural studies the difficulties of case definition are aggravated by the very differences that make such studies interesting, and are compounded by special problems in case finding and the collection of information. This chapter illustrates some of these problems by describing an attempt to explore the syndrome of childhood autism cross-culturally. The results of the study have been published elsewhere (Lotter, 1978), but will be referred to here to the extent that they usefully complement this methodological discussion.

The Syndrome

"Childhood autism" refers to a behavioral syndrome first described by Kanner in 1943. The essential behavioral features are: "a profound and general failure to develop social relationships; language retardation with impaired comprehension, echolalia and pronominal reversal; and ritualistic and compulsive phenomena" (Rutter, 1978, p. 4), with an onset within the first 2½ years of life. What has been learned about the syndrome in the 36 years since it was first described gives a clearer view of some of the remaining perplexities: there is great variability in intellectual level, in outcome, in specific behavioral features, in evidence of organic brain dysfunction, and in social background. The view that "some type of organic brain disorder" (Rutter, 1978) is involved is widely accepted, and no convincing evidence has been found that implicates psychological factors in etiology. Nevertheless, the epidemiologically confirmed excess of cases from middle-class homes remains unexplained, and we know that various forms of environmental intervention can be of benefit. Consequently the role of psychosocial influences of some kind cannot be dismissed, and it is an open question whether the syndrome may develop more readily, or differently, in different environments. We know that the syndrome appears in such ethnically diverse populations as Scandinavia and Japan; criteria for its recognition can be formulated so as to give roughly comparable rates of prevalence in studies done by different investigators in different countries (Wing et al., 1976), and we have some preliminary indications of possible risk factors. Since everything we know about autism comes from studies in industrialized, "developed" countries (however diverse in other ways) the most extreme cultural contrast may be afforded by "developing" countries.

Preliminary Questions

From this introductory discussion, three "problems" already arise. First, which "developing" country or region to explore? In our study we chose a region for investigation on practical grounds: language and cooperation. Sub-Saharan Africa includes a number of countries having in common a British colonial experience; in all of them English has been adopted as a professional and administrative language. Within this general region, preliminary contact by mail established those centers where sufficient cooperation would be forthcoming. Countries characterized at the time by excessive political turbulance were excluded from consideration.

Second, where the investigation attempted is a first effort, the epidemiologic question of prevalence must be approached in its most elementary form: does the syndrome occur at all? This question can have different meanings. In order to avoid the problems raised by "labeling" theory (Scheff, 1966; Waxler, 1977), the question was taken to mean "do the behaviors occur which in the West define the syndrome?" It cannot be assumed that classifications are cross-culturally valid. For example, Zemplini and Rabain (1965) have described a traditionally recognized abnormality in Senegal, with the local name of "nit-ku-bon." In a discussion of that work, Ellenberger (1968) has drawn attention to the similarity of the symptoms of some of the children included by this name, to those of autism as described in the West. However, the same name is applied also to children who are behaviorally very different. The point is that the basis for naming is different; the cultural *meaning* of the condition is primary, and can include widely diverse (to us) manifestations. The situation is analogous to the problems of classification often pointed out by anthropologists interested in cognition: that some societies may treat, say, an animal and a tree as members of the same class, apparently on the basis of totem membership. In short, we decided (as others have been obliged to do) simply to impose our own classification based on a Western point of view (e.g., German, 1972).

The third problem is a related one. Quite simply it is to find a way of answering the question often encountered when asking for cooperation or help: what's in it for us? That is, what is its local, practical relevance? The question has a certain point. The prevalence of mental illnesses generally, and relatively rare syndromes specifically, have no policy implications where mental health services are rudimentary and priority is given to an overwhelming frequency of treatable physical diseases. From that point of view Africa is not ready for psychiatric epidemiology (Sherwin and Schoelly, 1965). The same can be said for other developing regions (Carstairs, 1973; Leon, 1972; Neki, 1973). To ask for help with an investigation whose only relevance is to Western theoretical questions can strain hospitality. A different view sees any effort to understand mental disorder as having eventual universal relevance, since the "modernization" (Inkeles, 1969) of developing countries seems inevitable (Dubos, 1968). Moreover, recent studies are countering earlier views that psychological disorder is a "disease of civilization" (German, 1972); in some clinics in developing countries psychological disorders have been found to rival infectious diseases in frequency (Giel and van Luijk, 1969). Nevertheless, seeking cooperation in research which has no obvious practical relevance to immediate local concerns requires a certain delicacy of approach.

Where to Search? Finding a Population

If, then, the question is askable, the next issue concerns the area of search. How wide a net need be spread to find enough cases? In the autistic study two overriding facts decided the question. The first is the known rarity of the syndrome in developed countries (Lotter, 1966). Even in centers known to be interested in such problems, such as the Johns Hopkins Hospital in Baltimore, or the Hospital for Sick Children in London, an average of only about 7 or 8 new cases were seen in a year. Second, case finding depends on existing services having identified a population of handicapped children as possible cases. Such services, whether educational or medical, are not well developed in Africa. However, most countries in Africa have some provision for handicapped children. Blind or deaf children in Africa have long been served by charitable societies (Anderson, 1968), but attention is slowly being extended to include, for example, the mentally retarded. At the same time the absorption of independent schools and institutions into publicly funded and Government-run agencies has begun in a small way (UNESCO, 1974), mainly in the large urban centers. Consequently, in most large cities in Africa some aggregations of handicapped children can today be found. The obvious solution seemed therefore to sacrifice specificity of population in order to maximize the chances of case finding. In practice this meant visiting almost every major city in sub-Saharan Africa: Accra, Lagos, Ibadan (West Africa); Nairobi (East Africa); Lusaka, Salisbury (Central Africa); Johannesburg, Cape Town, Durban (Southern Africa).

Casting so wide a net in search of cases dilutes the meaning of what may be found by limiting comparison to an enormous, almost continental, conglomerate characterizable only in terms of the "traditional" cultures of these developing countries, and their economic poverty. For infrequently occurring disorders such as autism an extensive search is nevertheless essential. Recent attempts, using different methods, to assess the frequency of psychiatric disorder generally in African children illustrate the point. In his studies of children seen in an outpatient clinic in Uganda, Minde (1976, 1977) identified only two psychotic children; in the same country Egdell and Stanfield (1972) did not report any cases of psychosis among admissions to a neurology clinic. Neither Cederblad (1968), Baasher (1972), Giel et al. (1969), nor Nurcombe and Cawte (1967), in surveys of children in entire village populations in the Sudan, Ethiopia, and Carpentaria, respectively, reported any such cases. Even in more intensive local investigations, the tribal and linguistic diversity *within* the countries of Africa is an obstacle to the generalization of findings (Minde, 1975, German, 1972). We encountered an awkward practical illustration of these differences in a country of some 9 million people in which there were said to be many distinguishable language groups: speech therapy in the only large institution for the mentally retarded was therefore offered in English.

Locating and gaining access to identified congregations of handicapped children in the countries visited were practical problems requiring only persistence and energy. It may be helpful nevertheless to describe some of the difficulties that can be expected. All of them result in some way from the local expressions of the rapid social change characteristic of the entire region.

The extension of government involvement into the care of handicapped children is recent and seems to proceed in an ad hoc way. Government lists of facilities tend to be incomplete and unreliable. Often the informal guidance of government officials or officers of charitable societies is helpful, although sometimes limited by the transient incumbancy of ministry officials and conflicts associated with funding. Probably the most fruitful procedure is to identify one or two people whose *interest* in special care for children results in an acquaintance with various, sometimes informal, attempts to provide care. For example, we discovered through informal contacts an elderly, eccentric American lady in one city whose devoted care over many years for about 10 severely disordered young people in her own home, and whose ceaseless badgering of officials on their behalf, were widely known and admired, but were recorded in no official lists we could obtain. All these things arise against a background of official good intentions limited and frustrated by lack of money, lack of competent personnel, and confusion of purposes. Our access to what facilities there were was, however, always welcomed. We encountered a rather different situation in South Africa, where access to government-run mental institutions for African children was achieved only after very delicate and complicated negotiation through helpful intermediaries. The difficulties we encountered there were partly the consequence of recent "exposés" of conditions in the institutions by a quasi-religious group. It is now apparently illegal to describe conditions in such places without official consent. (In all fairness, and in contravention of that law, I have to say that the circumstances of the children I saw were comparable, in some instances favorably comparable, with those elsewhere in Africa.) Finally, although there is reason to suspect that autistic children might be found among groups of children with sensory handicaps such as deafness, the groups of this kind visited in the early part of the survey contained no behaviorally abnormal children. The reason evidently is that the limited numbers of places in these schools are eagerly sought, so that evidence of additional difficulties—retardation or behavior disorder, for example—results in a quick discharge to make room for a more promising or tractable candidate. Consequently, in later phases of the survey, searching for cases was limited to places known to contain mentally retarded children. At every stage however, any suggestion by individual medical or educational personnel that they "knew of" a specially "peculiar" child was followed up.

Case Finding

A population defined in this way has little epidemiologic usefulness for comparisons among the countries surveyed, but does provide a basis for gross comparison between developing and industrialized countries. This question is taken up later in the chapter. The next practical step was to screen the identified mentally handicapped children for possible cases of autism.

None of the various methods commonly used in the West was suitable by itself. Psychiatric diagnosis of autism in Western countries is not reliable between centers, and in Africa would be subject to undeterminable variability. There are few psychiatrists, and those there were had received their training in various schools in Europe or America. Elaborate checklists such as Rimland's E2 instrument (Rimland, 1971), intended to be completed by parents, are not useful with a largely illiterate population. Simple symptom checklists have been successfully employed in Africa to identify "behavior disorders" in normal school populations (Minde, 1975). More subtle judgments, however, are demanded for the identification of subgroups among abnormal children; the verbal interpretations needed are difficult even for native English speakers with wide experience of handicapped children. In Africa the ward and classroom personnel concerned with the mentally handicapped often have less formal education than regular school teachers so that an English language checklist would be inefficient and translation into the various local languages impractical.

A practical compromise was a methodologically crude but workable system of approximation, involving as a first step the rejection of all children for whom there was no suggestion from any source that they were possible cases. The sources of information and the basis for judgment can be described simply. Any child was retained if (a) in any case records, there appeared the labels "psychosis," "schizophrenia," or "autism," or any variant of them; (b) an informant used any of these terms verbally in describing a particular child; (c) case records or informants described any behavior corresponding to the main symptom categories of autism; (d) the writer observed such behavior. Finally, all children identified in this way were observed by the writer. These procedures repeated in all the centers visited produced 30 possible cases out of some 1300 children seen.

The aim in further examination of this group of 30 children was of course to select any who were comparable to those described in the West as autistic. The problem has two aspects: comparability of the symptoms themselves, and the combination of symptoms into a comparable syndrome.

The Symptoms

The paucity of good developmental histories is a major problem. (Much of the detailed description of autistic symptoms offered by Kanner, for example, was derived from what parents had observed and reported to him.) The characteristic similarity of autistic children dissipates somewhat with age, especially after about 5 years. Moreover, without a description of early development, an estimate of the probable age of onset is impossible. The problem is common to any study of autism, but was grossly exaggerated in the countries we explored, for several interrelated reasons. Even for serious physical disease, children in Africa are usually brought to hospitals or clinics "too late" (Goodall, 1972; Godel, 1971), and none of our 30 possible cases was younger than 7 years old. Case records are generally very poor, with scanty details about developmental histories. In part this seems to be the result of inadequate recording, and in part, the poverty of information available to the examining physician from the parents (Egdell and Stanfield, 1972). Quite often members of the extended family other than the parents will accompany the child, and they may be ignorant of the developmental information asked for. Language problems may be met by using interpreters; but the three-part conceptual struggle between the Western doctor, his indigenous but westernized interpreter, and the patient (plus supporting relatives) is rich in possibilities for misunderstanding. Giel et al. (1969) describe the situation like this:

> Interpreters, especially if they are trained in medicine, tend to be very selective in their translations. They look for what they consider to be medically relevant, and leave out all the rest of a patient's statements. They feel embarrassed or they become ironical when a patient tries to express himself in his own words, and uses his own familiar images. One can, for example, observe from his gestures how a patient hesitates as to where to localize his symptoms, while using the word *lib* (heart). The interpreter, wanting to get on with his job and relying on previous experience, decides that the complaints are "epigastric". From then on it is almost impossible to learn more about this patient's true feelings. Moreover, patients do not just state their complaints but dramatize them, supported by a clear interaction with their often many and deeply interested companions. (P. 158)

It is not easy to see how the difficulties in eliciting and interpreting symptom descriptions and developmental histories can be overcome by an expatriate researcher. Descriptions of referral complaints about young children suggest that a failure to achieve an expected level of development generally, or specifically in walking and talking, and fits, are most common (Egdell and Stanfield, 1972). These complaints can perhaps be taken as some indication of early abnormality least subject to problems of interpretation. Even with the reports of fits however there may be reason for caution; breath-holding, for example, may be reported as epilepsy (Nurcombe and Cawte, 1967).

For all these reasons case recognition in our study relied very little on the history, and mostly on our own observations of present behavior or on descriptions of postreferral development obtained from institution personnel.

Special problems in the recognition of individual symptoms arose partly as a consequence of the kind of population being explored, and partly from the cultural context. Most of the children we saw were mentally retarded, many to a severe degree. Among the 30 selected children most did not speak at all, and few of the rest had better than very limited speech. In the absence of reliable information about whether the mute children had ever spoken, the usefulness of the "speech" symptom category was limited to a recording of the muteness, and in the few speaking children, echolalia and a noncommunicative repetition of simple phrases. For any cross-cultural study attempting to include less severely handicapped autistic children, the recognition of the peculiar *uses* of speech, described at length by Kanner (1946) would provide a fascinating challenge. In the four speaking children we saw who were not also severely subnormal, we could find no evidence of the kinds of speech use Kanner described—but to recognize them in a strange language through informants is not easy.

The other two main symptoms—social "aloneness" and what we called a class of repetitive ritualistic behaviors assumed therefore an additional importance for case recognition. In combination we used them in a previous study (Lotter, 1967) to define a subgroup of autistic children that seemed most closely to resemble Kanner's Syndrome. In that study the repetitive ritualistic phenomena seemed especially to distinguish a core subgroup from other less markedly autistic children who also were severely impaired socially. In Africa we found it no more difficult than in the British study to rate the items in the "social" category. It seems likely that attempts to discover evidence of abnormal social behavior in infants by questioning mothers will run into the sorts of difficulties described by Giel and his colleagues. Little seems to be known about traditional expectations about normal development, or tolerance of deviance.

To apply Western developmental expectations cross-culturally may be misleading. For example, the passivity of Ghanaian young children (Bain, 1973) might be considered deviant in North America; Kagan and Klein (1973) expressed surprise at the developmental "recovery" of apparently retarded infants in Guatemala; and quite generally Western preoccupations with explicit criteria of normal development have been said to puzzle informants in China (Kessen, 1975).

There are few difficulties in recognizing instances of the peculiarities of movement and manipulation of, or preoccupation with, objects that constitute the third class of phenomena. They are at the same time most readily visible, and easily described to an informant, if necessary by imitation. We were surprised therefore at how few instances we found of this kind of behavior, both in our direct observations and in informants' reports. Examples of nonfunctional collecting of objects, the "inappropriate use of toys," or a peculiar fascination with mechanical things, which often illustrate aspects of this symptom in Western experience, may be rare in Africa simply because cardboard boxes, toys, and mechanical gadgets are less ubiquitously available. On the other hand, very simple forms of these activities, such as carrying often a stick or leaf, or banging simple objects repetitively, were not uncommon in Africa. There seemed, from our own observation and from reports to us, also to be much less gross stereotypic rocking and head banging than is commonly found in Western institutions. Each of these broad classes of behavior requires detailed study in order to resolve the questions about the form and frequency of their occurrence in developing countries raised here.

Summarizing so far, we have argued that as the Western practice of extending institutionalized forms of care to chronically handicapped children expands in the developing regions of Africa the resulting congregations of children form an increasing pool of readily available subjects for cross-cultural study. Because of economic factors, local priorities, shortage of trained personnel, as well as language and other cultural differences, clinical records are of very limited usefulness. Developmental histories depending on parents are likely to be even less reliable in developing countries than in the West. While the behavioral discrimination of abnormal children may be achieved through the use of teacher-rated questionnaires, direct observation is necessary for distinctions *among* handicapped children.

The Syndrome

There is no unique description of childhood autism which accommodates the many differences among individual children who exhibit "autistic behavior." Apart from the age of onset, there is no special problem in defining the behavioral syndrome of autism in cross-cultural material, once the elements have been established. Of the various ways this can be done, we chose the simplest: rating each item for presence and severity, ranking cases according to total "symptom score," and selecting of an arbitrary cutoff point, distinguishing between those cases with "more" autistic behavior (whom we called autistic) and those with less. The procedure was similar to one we had used previously for a survey in Britain (Lotter, 1967) with whose results we hoped to make some comparisons. In this way we defined a group of nine African children as autistic, and a residual group as "not autistic." These "not autistic" children had for a variety of reasons been judged to be possible cases at an earlier stage of screening.

We could say, then, that behavioral elements of the syndrome of childhood autism do occur in African populations, and that the elements co-occur in individual children who, according to a symptom-accumulation definition, could be said to exhibit the syndrome. Although to that extent behaviorally similar, the children in the group were in many other ways heterogeneous. Three aspects of this heterogeneity may be useful in the comparison of groups of autistic children: intellectual level, evidence of "brain damage," and social background. Any attempt to describe these characteristics faces special problems in cross-cultural work. It is important to consider them since a "triaxial" system which incorporates these three aspects has been proposed for child psychiatric classification generally (Rutter et al., 1969).

Intellectual Level

Some consideration of intellectual functioning in autistic children is necessary because the interpretation of symptoms must be appropriate to mental age (Rutter, 1978; Wing and Gould, 1979) and because etiological factors may be different for autistic children of normal or near-normal intelligence in contrast to those who appear severely retarded. Moreover, careful testing often reveals a selective retardation in verbal skills. Until locally standardized testing instruments are developed for African conditions only gross estimates of intellectual level are possible, and no useful comparisons can be made of patterns of functioning.

Most of our cases were found among children already recognized as mentally subnormal, usually severely subnormal. In Western groups of autistic children about one-quarter are not additionally handicapped by serious mental retardation. When young, they, as well as some who eventually turn out to be severely subnormal, may seem to be merely odd, and even precocious in some respects. At one time Kanner insisted that autistic children were intellectually normal. Few of these less severely handicapped children could appear in our survey. One of the reasons is the tendency in Africa for psychological abnormality to be interpreted somatically (Giel et al., 1969). Illness is organic illness. There are few direct complaints about "emotional" disorders (Egdell and Stanfield, 1972), and "behavior disorders" are seldom seen in clinics. According to Minde (1976) such problems in children are dealt with simply by expulsion from school, or punishment. These observations from Uganda are closely parallelled by those of Singer et al. (1978) in Hong Kong. Consequently cases of autism least complicated by mental retardation which represent in some ways the most interesting group for sociocultural comparison, are least likely to appear in identified groups of handicapped children in developing countries. It is among this subgroup that the most important observations concerning the possible role of cultural factors in determining the course of the disorder, and the occurrence and patterning of symptoms, remain to be made. In what way these kinds of observations will be possible depends largely on how the conceptual and methodological questions surrounding the measurement of intelligence in traditional societies are resolved (Serpell, 1972).

Social Background

One of the most curious aspects of childhood autism in Western countries is the frequently reported excess of educated middle-class parents. Over 90% of Kanner's cases came from "professional" families (Kanner and Lesser, 1958). Epidemiologic surveys have shown that this is a real difference in prevalence not explainable by selective referral (Lotter, 1967), although the difference is less marked than Kanner's figures suggested. No satisfactory explanation for the finding has been offered, nor has good evidence been found which implicates parental personality or attitude characteristics as causative factors (Cantwell et al., 1978). Asking the question in Africa raised two problems: the definition of "social class," and the possible selective use of social services.

Social class in Western societies may be defined by occupation, as in Britain, where there are population statistics routinely collected which offer a basis for comparison; or by composite indices such as the Hollingshead (1958) scale of socioeconomic status. In Africa there are no comparable population statistics, and although Western SES scales are sometimes used there (Minde, 1977), they are not generally appropriate. According to Lloyd (1966), the small "elite" groups in Africa, while defined by education and consequent privilege, are not comparable to a Western class stratification. Unlike Western classes which may be characterized by shared attitudes, child-rearing patterns, patterns of family life and so on, African elites cut across tribal (and therefore local cultural) affiliations. Moreover, it has been shown that formal education is not inconsistent with the retention of traditional attitudes and beliefs (Jahoda, 1968; Bain, 1973; Lloyd, 1966). The common factor between African elite groups and Western autistic children's families is relative superiority in formal education. Apart from being more readily available, this index was useful for our study since in the absence of population statistics, a comparison could be made between the autistic and nonautistic cases. Since formal education implies in Africa a privileged exposure to Western culture, we expanded the definition of "education" to include other forms of similar exposure, such as having lived in a Western industrial country.

All this was of course very rough-and-ready categorizing. But we were especially interested in the question of social class because in Longe and Asuni's (1972) Nigerian report, the parents of *all* their 4 autistic cases were University graduates or had studied abroad, or both. The most obvious explanation of their astonishing finding was selective use of psychiatric services by the elite class. The authors consider this, but report that "the large majority" of the parents using the clinic "are illiterate or have low levels of academic attainment." A similar account of attendance at a Lagos pediatric clinic (Gans, 1963), and a dissenting finding in Uganda (Minde, 1977) leave the question of selective use of facilities unclear. Possibly different patterns of referral occur in different places. What is agreed, however, is that education does not lead to an abandonment of belief in and consultation of traditional healers (Jahoda, 1968; Neki, 1973; Bain, 1973; Twumasi, 1975; Lambo, 1961; Olatawura, 1978, Boroffka and Olatawura, 1977). Membership in the "elite" does not by itself distinguish a pattern of use of public services—the privileged and the poor use both traditional and modern medical and social services. Examination of our own data showed that while about 63% of our possible cases had "elite" families, the proportion among the autistic cases was larger (78%) than in the nonautistic comparison group (58%). Thus, on the face of it, in Africa as in the West the kinds of behavior called autistic seem to be associated with the level of formal education in the families of index cases.

"Brain Damage"

The role of neurological disorder in the etiology of autism is not clear; in some cases there is good evidence of cerebral dysfunction, especially where there is also mental retardation. In others no such evidence can be found. Others again may develop fits for the first time in adolescence, in the absence of previous evidence of neurological disorder. Specification of such evidence is important in continuing attempts at classification. Our question was whether the general findings for autism were repeated in an African group. Because the diagnosis of "brain damage" can be uncertain even with the best facilities (Rutter, 1977), and refined neurological examination of children is not usual in Africa, we limited our observations to recorded presence of epilepsy.

Direct comparison with Western groups is inappropriate for two main reasons. First, the background circumstances are different: according to Egdell and Stanfield (1972) children in (tropical) developing countries "are exposed to more frequent environmental hazards, such as birth trauma, acquired infection, malnutrition, hyperthermia, and water and electrolyte disturbances." They go on to speak of the "vast background of feverish illness in children presenting at out-patient departments and rural dispensaries . . ." Moreover, "late or ineffective treatment of these conditions adds to the toll of brain damaged children among the survivors while the introduction of effective treatment of formerly killing diseases inevitably results in the survival of an increasing number of damaged individuals" (p. 548). Secondly, there are strongly held beliefs about epilepsy in all parts of Africa (Egdell and Stanfield, 1972; Sinnette, 1970; German, 1972; Giel et al., 1969). Generally these involve the idea that the disorder is contagious, so that epileptics may be shunned. For this reason (adult) epileptics have little chance of appearing in household *or* in school surveys (Anderson, 1968; Giel et al., 1969). At the same time, secondary hazards of epilepsy are evident, such as in some of the consequences of traditional treatments (e.g., burning the feet) (Oluwasanmi, 1973).

These are profound cultural differences likely to influence the incidence of epilepsy and the frequency with which epileptics will be discovered. It seemed reasonable in our own study to compare the African autistic and nonautistic groups, since both would presumably have been subject to similar selective factors. Somewhat to our surprise, we found a pattern similar to that in Western groups, that is, relatively more epilepsy among the autistic children with less-marked symptoms, relatively more epilepsy among the severely retarded autistic children, and relatively more epilepsy among the nonautistic comparison group. While these findings can be interpreted variously, they do show that the picture of the relation between autistic behavior and neurological disorder appears in Africa in a way that is not remarkably different from that in the West.

Prevalence

The cases identified in our autistic survey obviously cannot be the basis for any statement about prevalence in any of the countries visited, nor for Africa as a whole. Even where case finding is more thorough and confined to single centers or local communities, a prevalence rate of psychiatric morbidity cannot be generalized confidently because of the ethnic and cultural diversity within and among African countries (Giel et al., 1969; Minde, 1977; German, 1972).

It seemed worth asking instead, whether autism occurs among the severely subnormal in Africa with a frequency comparable to that in Western countries. The problem of ethnic and cultural diversity is not solved, but may be said to be partly avoided by defining both index cases and population at risk as severely and chronically abnormal (Edgerton, 1969). The comparison is thus restricted to individuals who would probably be considered abnormal in any society. In Britain between 5 and 8% of severely subnormal children are autistic (Lotter, 1967). The corresponding proportion in our African data is about 2½%. Why is this? Infantile death is common is Africa (Morley, 1963; Godel, 1971; Gulbinat and Ernberg, 1978) but are autistic infants more likely to die than other severely subnormal children? Perhaps because of socially disruptive behavior they are more readily abandoned by their families to become part of the child-flotsam of Africa described by Minde (1977). He speaks of children who had lost the support of their extended families "wandering through the country from age 7 onwards, living off the land, being exploited and mishandled until they were finally picked up by the police . . ." (p. 32). It has been suggested that feral children may be abandoned autistic children (Bettelheim, 1967). Yet we saw too many nonautistic children whose disordered behavior might have been expected to have attracted to them a similar fate. Perhaps the ubiquitous extended family found a way to live with them? Yet the tolerance of the extended family may not extend so readily to *troublesome* subnormal children (Egdell and Stanfield, 1972). Singer et al. (1978) have even argued that the extended family structure may exacerbate behavior problems through, for example, a diffusion of authority. It may be that African autistic children have less disruptive behavior and so come less often to administrative attention. The traditional *meaning* given to the "nit-ku-bon" child in Senegal would seem to preclude his being abandoned, even into an institution, and the management of his peculiarities predicated upon that interpretation might be expected to minimize his disruptive influence. The Wolof believe the "nit-ku-bon" child does not speak and is socially unresponsive because he is a rare soul highly developed through many incarnations and can therefore be expected to find spiritually inferior persons uncongenial. His superior development reasonably accounts for his irritation at being treated as a child; what we call tantrums are therefore treated as inconvenient emotional outbursts which are understandable reactions to inappropriate management. An appropriate response is to defer to his desires, and to avoid frustrating him in any way.

We encountered no accounts of comparable beliefs among informants elsewhere in Africa. The fact remains that we found some autisticlike children in each of the centers we visited, and in aggregate fewer than we thought we should have found.

Conclusion

There is a dilemma at the heart of cross-cultural psychiatric research, perhaps even a paradox. There are two kinds of reasons for asking cross cultural questions, reasons of practical utility as in the provision of services, and reasons of scientific understanding. The paradox lies in this: utility assumes modernization, and modernization destroys the contrast that is the peculiar virtue of cross-cultural study. Putting it another way, "traditional" societies are merely backward versions of our own unless they represent also interestingly different ways of thinking. Imposing our own scientific conceptions of experience blinds us to the differences that define and justify cross-cultural research.

Thus, from the point of view of utility, Africa may not be "ready" for epidemiologic research. Presumably it will become ready when its societies more closely resemble our own in administrative efficiency (more reliable statistics and records) and institutional structure (for using the results of research in organizing prevention, treatment, and disposition of unfit people). And by then much of what is meant by, and valuable in, the idea of cross-cultural research may be gone.

The dilemma seems most acute in research into adult disorders where symptoms involve reports of subjective experience, like hallucinations (Al-Issa, 1977). It appears in another form in investigations of childhood behavior disorders, such as those of Minde in Kampala, where assessments are made by teachers and parents according to Western categories of deviance. The dilemma is of course well known in anthropology, and in a different way, in history. Psychological disorders of children may be least subject to these problems of interpretation, especially where the disorders are severe and chronic, as in autism which is capable of reasonably reliable description. If this is true, then the main problems are practical ones of data collection, and it is with these that this chapter has been most concerned.

Four practical issues stand out. The first is the question of developmental histories which for descriptions of onset and course are of special importance in autism. The second concerns the severity of handicap. Nearly all the children we saw were severely subnormal; what is needed is some way of discovering autistic children in Africa who are not also severely handicapped intellectually, and who are not readily brought to attention within the services as presently developed in Africa. The third relates to the urban bias of our sample. Most people in developing countries do not live in cities, and are more closely connected still with the traditional culture. We need to know whether, and in what way autism develops in rural villages. Finally, we do not know what the long-term course of autism may be in Africa, especially the outcome for autistic children who are not severely subnormal. We assume from Western studies that autism is chronically disabling. Whether more transient forms occur, as are reported for schizophrenia in recent cross-cultural studies (Sartorius et al., 1978) is a question of obvious importance in relation to etiology.

All these issues lend themselves to, perhaps even demand, indigenously based research. Most of the problems we have raised are tractable, and could be readily addressed within the broader context of the developing network of general pediatric services in Africa.

References

Al-Issa, I. Social and cultural aspects of hallucinations. Psych. Bull., 84, 1977, 570–587.

Anderson, E. M. *The Education of Physically Handicapped Blind and Deaf Children in East Africa.* London, National Foundation for Research in Crippling Diseases, 1968.

Baasher, T. A. Childhood psychiatric disorders in the Sudan. Paper read at Third Pan-African Psychiatric Conference, Khartoum, 1972.

Bain, S. E. Childhood socialization in 20 educated families in Accra. MSc. Thesis, University of Guelph, 1973.

Bettelheim, B. *The Empty Fortress.* New York, Free Press, 1967.

Boroffka, A. and Olatawura, M. O. Community psychiatry in Nigeria—the current status. Comm. Psychiat., 23, 1977, 275–281.

Cantwell, D. P., Baker, L., and Rutter, M. Family Factors. In M. Rutter and E. Schopler (Eds.) *Autism: A Reappraisal of Concepts and Treatment.* New York, Plenum, 1978.

Carstairs, G. M. Psychiatric problems of developing countries. Brit. J. Psychiat., 123, 1973, 271–277.

Cederblad, M. A child psychiatric study of Sudanese Arab children. Acta Psychiat. Scand. (Suppl.) 200, 1968, 1–230.

Dubos, R. *Man, Medicine and Environment.* New York, Praeger, 1968.

Edgerton, R. B. On the "recognition" of mental illness. In S. Plog and R. B. Edgerton (Eds.) *Changing Perspectives in Mental Illness.* New York, Holt, 1969.

Egdell, H. G. and Stanfield, J. P. Paediatric neurology in Africa: a Ugandan report. Brit. med. J., 1, 1972, 548–552.

Ellenberger, H. F. Impressions psychiatriques d'un sejour a Dakar. Canad. Psychiat. Ass. J., 13, 1968, 539–549.

Gans, B. Some socio-economic and cultural factors in West African pediatrics. Arch. Dis. Child., 38, 1963, 1–12.

German, G. A. Aspects of clinical psychiatry in sub-Saharan Africa, Brit. J. Psychiat., 121, 1972, 461–479.

Giel, R. and van Luijk, J. N. Psychiatric morbidity in a small Ethiopian town. Brit. J. Psychiat., 115, 1969, 149–162.

Giel, R., Bishaw, M., and van Luijk, J. N. Behaviour disorders in Ethiopian children. Psychiat. Neurol. Neurochir., 72, 1969, 395–400.

Godel, J. C. A paediatric tragedy. Medilag, 1, 1971, 8–9.

Goodall, J. (Ed.) The hospital care of East African children. Env. Child Hlth., 18, 1972, 45–125.

Graham, P. J. Epidemiological issues and child psychiatry. Int. J. Ment. Hlth., 7, 1978, 6–23.

Gulbinat, W. and Ernberg, G. Demographic considerations and trends. Int. J. Ment. Hlth., 7, 1978, 18–33.

Inkeles, A. Making men modern: On the causes and consequences of individual change in six developing countries. Amer. J. Sociol., 75, 1969, 208–225.

Jahoda, G. Scientific training and the persistence of traditional beliefs among West African university students. Nature, 220, 1968.

Kagan, J. and Klein, R. E. Cross-cultural perspectives on early development. Amer. Psychol., 28, 1973, 1356.

Kanner, L. Autistic disturbances of affective contact. Nerv. Child., 2, 1943, 217–250.

Kanner, L. Irrelevant and metaphonical language in early infantile autism. Amer. J. Psychiat., 103, 1946, 242–246.

Kanner, L. and Lesser, L. I. Early infantile autism. Ped. Clin. N. Amer., 5, 1958, 711–730.

Kessen, W. (Ed.) *Childhood in China.* New Haven, Yale University Press, 1975.

Lambo, T. A. Growth of African children. Paper read at First Pan-African Congress on Mental Health, Abeokuta, 1961.

Leon, C. A. Psychiatry in Latin America. Brit. J. Psychiat., 121, 1972, 121–136.

Lloyd, B. B. Education and family life in the development of class identification among the Yoruba. In P. C. Lloyd (Ed.) *The New Elites of Tropical Africa.* London, Oxford University Press, 1966.

Longe, C. I. and Asuni, T. Four cases of infantile autism in Nigerian children. Paper read at Third Pan-African Psychiatric Conference, Khartoum, 1972.

Lotter, V. Epidemiology of autistic conditions in young children: prevalence. Soc. Psychiat., 1, 1966, 124–137.

Lotter, V. Epidemiology of autistic conditions in young children: some characteristics of the parents and children. Soc. Psychiat., 1, 1967, 163–173.

Lotter, V. Childhood autism in Africa. J. Child Psychol. Psychiat., 19, 1978, 231–244.

Minde, K. K. Psychological problems in Ugandan school children: a controlled evaluation. J. Child Psychol. Psychiat., 16, 1975, 49–59.

Minde, K. K. Child psychiatry in developing countries. J. child Psychol. Psychiat., 17, 1976, 79–83.

Minde, K. K. Child psychiatry in developing countries. J. Child Psychol. Psychiat., 17, 1976, 79–83.

Minde, K. K. Children in Uganda: rates of behavioural deviations and psychiatric disorders in various school and clinic populations. J. Child Psychol. Psychiat., 18, 1977, 23–27.

Morley, P. A medical service for children under 5 years of age in West Africa. J. Trop. Med. and Hygiene, 57, 1963, 79–88.

Neki, J. S. Psychiatry in South-east Asia. Brit. J. Psychiat., 123, 1973, 257–269.

Nurcombe, B. and Cawte, J. E. Patterns of behaviour disorder amongst the children of an aboriginal population. Aust. N. Z. J. Psychiat, 1, 1967, 119–133.

Olatawura, M. O. Mental health services for children in the African region. Int. J. Ment. Hlth., 7, 1978, 34–38.

Oluwasanmi, J. O. Burns of the feet. Nigerian med J., 3, 1973, 146–148.

Rimland, B. The differentiation of childhood psychosis: an analysis of checklists for 2218 psychotic children. J. Aut. Child Schiz., 1, 1971, 161–174.

Rutter, M., Lebovici, S., Eisenberg, L., Sneznevskij, A. V., Sadoun, R., Brooke, E. and Lin, T-Y. A tri-axial classification of mental disorders in childhood. J. Child Psychol. Psychiat., 10, 1969, 41–61.

Rutter, M. Diagnosis and Definition. In M. Rutter and E. Schopler, (Eds.) *Autism: A Reappraisal of Concepts and Treatment*, New York, Plenum, 1978.

Rutter, M. Brain damage syndromes in childhood: concepts and findings. J. Child Psychol. Psychiat., 18, 1977, 1–21.

Sartorius, N., Jablensky, A., and Shapino, R. Cross-cultural differences in the short-term prognosis of schizophrenic psychoses. Schiz. Bull., 4, 1978, 102–113.

Scheff, T. *Being Mentally Ill.* Chicago, Aldine, 1966.

Serpell, R. Aspects of intelligence in a developing country, Afr. Soc. Res., 17, 1972, 578–596.

Sherwin, A. C. and Schoelly, M. L. Criteria of Psychiatric disorder in children. In J. M. Murphy and A. H. Leighton, (Eds) *Approaches to Cross-Cultural Psychiatry,* Cornell, Cornell University Press, 1965.

Singer, K., Ney, P. G., and Lieh-Mak, F. A cultural perspective on child psychiatric disorders. Comp. Psychiat., 19, 1978, 533–540.

Sinnette, C.H. The handicapped child in tropical Africa. Courrier, 20, 1970, 335–345.

Twumasi, P. A. *Medical Systems in Ghana: a Study in Medical Sociology*. Accra, Ghana Publishing Co., 1975.

Unesco. *Case Studies in Special Education*. Paris, The Unesco Press, 1974.

Waxler, N. F. Is mental illness cured in traditional societies? A theoretical analysis. Culture, Med. Psychiat., 1, 1977, 233–253.

Wing, L., and Gould, J. Systematic recording of behaviors and skills of retarded and psychotic children. (Univ. London Inst. of Psychiatry, England) J. of Autism and Childhood Schizophrenia, 1978 (Mar.) Vol 8 (1) 79–97.

Wing, L., Yeates, S. R., Brierley, L. M., and Gould, J. The prevalence of early childhood autism: A comparison of administrative and epidemiological studies. Psych. Med. 6, 1976, 89–100.

Zemplini, A., and Rabain, J. L'enfant nit-ku-bon. Un tableaux psychopathologique traditionnel chez Les Wolof et Lebou du Senegal. Psychopath. Afr., 1, 1965, 329–441.

Theory and Method in Child Psychiatric Epidemiology

SHEPPARD G. KELLAM, M.D.

MARGARET E. ENSMINGER, PH.D.

Epidemiology is the study of the distribution and causes of disease or disorder in total, defined populations. In child psychiatry, epidemiology can have at least three purposes. The first is understanding the origins and course of child psychiatric illness or disorder. A second is understanding the significance of early circumstances, events, behavior, and disorder in the evolving life course of the individual. The third is providing baseline and outcome information about the needs of the disturbed children in a total population for the design and evaluation of intervention programs.

Among the highly insular social, behavioral, and biological sciences in America, psychiatric epidemiology has been peculiarly separate as a discipline. However, it is becoming increasingly important as a function of almost all of the different disciplines which are interested in the origins and course of mental health and illness. Recently, as this volume attests, increasing attention has been paid to child psychiatric epidemiologic research.

The relation of theory to method in child psychiatric epidemiology is problematic in several ways: many question the reliability and validity of clinical assessments done in large numbers outside of the clinical examining room, often by less trained interviewers. There is a lack of consensus regarding definitions of mental health and illness, and the kind of theory best suited to uncovering the etiology of child disorders. These and other problems leave many pessimistic about the future of epidemiology in child psychiatry. It is our purpose in this paper to show how the clarification of central concepts can help.

The most useful first approach, given this situation, is to find that centrally important problem area which, if advanced, will allow alternative theories and methods to evolve and be tested. It is our thesis—and therefore the focus of this chapter—that the first step is to identify certain theoretical constructs without which theory can neither be built nor tested.

Concepts such as mental health system, patient status, community, family, mental health, and mental illness are all central to using epidemiologic methods for exploring and testing theory in child psychiatry. These constructs are disarmingly simple at first glance, but we will attempt to demonstrate here that research has been severely hampered by the lack of clarity and detail as to their meaning and their measurement. We propose to examine each construct, not exhaustively, but describing essential aspects of each and illustrating how we have approached their measurement in the Woodlawn mental health studies. These longitudinal, prospective, community epidemiologic child psychiatric studies were conducted in an urban, poor, black community on the South Side of Chicago. We investigated four consecutive total populations of first-grade children periodically from first to third grades, including assessments of the families of two of the cohorts and a 10-year follow-up of one total cohort.

Longitudinal research is an essential strategy in epidemiology and offers a partial solution to some of the problems noted above. However, a longitudinal approach can also create its own problems. Evolving age, changing societal context, and idiosyncratic significant life events all may influence behavior or disorder in important ways; they also present problems of measurement, design, and interpretation (Baltes et al., 1980). We will address selected aspects of these problems in the context of discussing the above-mentioned theoretical constructs.

Epidemiology entails investigating causes of illness or disorder by examining conditions associated with variation in incidence and prevalence, both concurrently and over time. It is not frequently associated with the experimental method, which could add great strength to epidemiologic research. Community-wide prevention or early intervention studies, if defined on the basis of theoretically important hypotheses, can be an important and effective quasi-experimental model for studying the validity of aspects of theory. Such epidemiologic quasi experiments have not often been done in child psychiatry, but the Woodlawn first-grade prevention and early intervention study is an example of such a community-wide quasi experiment (Kellam et al., 1975). The purpose of the first-grade program was to improve the adequacy of the social task performance of the first graders in six of the 12 Woodlawn schools. The two groups of six schools were matched and a flip of a coin determined which were intervention and which control. The study was repeated in three consecutive first-grade cohorts.

The theoretical question we were asking was, what was the

evolving relationship between psychological well-being (PWB) and performance on the social tasks the teacher required of the children, as assessed by the teacher. We have named this kind of rating social adaptational status (SAS). This quasi experiment in prevention tested whether by improving social task performance the children's concurrent and later PWB would improve also. The six matched control schools served as a base for comparison.

Social adaptational status was improved modestly but consistently in the six intervention schools at least as far as third grade. While the overall level of PWB remained the same in the intervention and control schools, the relationship between the SAS and PWB increased in the intervention schools; that is, children who performed better in intervention schools had better PWB by clinical ratings and self-reports than their counterparts in control schools. However, children in intervention schools who performed poorly had more risk of psychological symptoms than their counterparts in control schools. Our interpretation of this finding was that, by concentrating on improving classroom performance, the first-grade program may have increased the psychological significance of the classroom tasks. We are now analyzing the significance of these results 10 years later and will report on early analyses in our discussion of mental health and illness.

These results confirmed the relationship in Woodlawn between teacher-assessed classroom task performance and PWB from first to third grade, and also indicated some of the complex characteristics of the relationship. Such epidemiologic intervention quasi experiments often can be done with benefit to program design as well as to theory, by providing specific baseline assessments and evaluation of the impact of the intervention program.

Sociology, psychology, psychiatry, education, and a variety of other sciences concerned with mental health and illness all can make important theoretical and methodological contributions to how epidemiologic research questions are framed and how the research is to be designed. Epidemiology, in turn, offers an orientation, a core of useful constructs, and analytic methods for examining variation in defined populations concurrently and longitudinally.

Our focus on theoretical constructs begins with an examination of how epidemiology fits into an overall framework for understanding research and service in mental health and illness. We have called this first conceptual issue the "mental health system." By beginning here, we wish to underline epidemiologic research's concern with total populations, healthy as well as ill. Populations of only ill or disordered people found in outpatient clinics or hospitals comprise different denominators than the populations of both healthy and ill required in epidemiologic studies.

The Mental Health System

We have found it useful to envision a mental health system in which there are three levels. The first is highly integrated into the local community and includes those aspects of service and research related to prevention, early treatment, and many aspects of continued treatment. This level has a community focus. The concern is with total populations of healthy and ill, and with the cultural, social, and political structure of the community. Epidemiologic research is centered in this level of the mental health system.

Studies at this level often require considerable involvement in the social and political contexts of the community both for access to individuals and social fields and for developing and maintaining the support of citizens. An old public health adage holds that only if you persuade the key person in a community to take the vaccine will the rest of the community take it. This still holds true in many communities and is a typical problem for both research and service at the first level (see Kellam et al., 1972; Kellam and Branch, 1971).

The second level is more specialized and occurs in more traditional outpatient settings, such as the private practitioner's office or the mental health clinic of the local hospital. The essential characteristic of this level is the concern with outpatient populations already in need.

The third level of the mental health system consists of hospital and its variations. At this level the population requiring extensive specialized professional care is served, and relevant research in such areas is carried on. Typically, the third level would serve a much broader geographic area than the first (which is related to a single neighborhood) and a more disturbed population than either the second or the first.

Epidemiologic research can be and has been done on second and third level populations, but such studies require extreme care in matching healthy controls with the ill populations which make up second- and third-level denominators. Such case-control studies are prone to problems in matching and make it difficult to include in the research the social characteristics of a specific community area. Disorders which are very infrequent can sometimes only be studied using this research model. Whenever possible, community epidemiology is usually preferable since it allows for more specific and extensive control populations. It also provides more opportunity for the study of community, family, school, peers, and the interplay of these with biological variables, as part of hypothesized causes or influences on health, illness, or disorder.

This view of a mental health system implies a high order of integration across the three levels, with the first level permitting the kinds of research and service which follow from the close relationship to populations of healthy as well as ill individuals. It is here that epidemiologic research is centrally important as a way of studying the amounts, kinds and determinants of clinical states and growth and development. It is also important in providing a baseline for the development, study, and evaluation of prevention, early intervention, and treatment programs. The second and third levels focus on populations already in need and therefore cannot function in primary prevention; prevention at these two levels is restricted to alleviating morbidity.

Who Becomes a Patient and the Mental Health System—The fundamental differences between the three levels of this mental health system concept are the different denominators which comprise the population of each level. The first-level denominator consists of the total population in a defined community area. The second consists of those who have come to outpatient clinic facilities, and the third consists of those in need of hospital or its variations. The flow of people across these three levels is not yet well understood. Often, psychiatric research is based on the assumption that the patients in the second or third level represent the ill part of the first-level population. Little or no evidence exists to confirm this assumption. In the Woodlawn studies of why teenagers come to treatment, for example, no evidence was found of a relationship between distress and seeking help. Other studies we will cite below also point to a wide array of reasons other than illness or disorder which influence help-seeking behavior.

As part of the 10-year follow-up of the 1966-67 Woodlawn first graders, a treatment program was designed which included such services as psychotherapy, remedial reading and mathematics, vocational counseling, group discussion sessions, and a variety of other activities directed at the wide range of adolescent psychosocial needs.

Pairs of black college students conducted the 10-year follow-up assessment sessions, which included five to eight Woodlawn teenagers at a session. One of the assessors was primary, with the other in a secondary role. At the beginning of the sessions, the two assessors led a group discussion with the teenagers concerning reasons for asking questions in such personal areas as family, peer group involvement, drug use, and PWB.

Our hypothesis was that teenagers who came for help would have more early and concurrent psychological distress, problems in social fields such as school, peer group, the family, and/or with the police. The results showed that none of these problems seemed to influence teenagers to come into the treatment program. Seeking help was a function of the particular primary assessor who happened to be carrying out the assessment sessions. The same assessor in the secondary role had no such effect. Figure 1 shows each assessor's record regarding the percent of teenagers he or she assessed who came for an initial treatment interview. Each bar represents one assessor, the left side when that assessor was in the primary role, the right when in the secondary role. We can see from this figure that when one assessor was in the primary role, over 50% of the teenagers came in for at least an intake interview. The same assessor in the secondary role showed no such dramatic difference from his or her colleagues. When other assessors were in the primary role, remarkably few teenagers came for intake, with the figure for one assessor being as low as 5% (Kellam et al., 1980b).

FIGURE 1

Effects of Assessors
in Primary and Secondary
Roles on Teenagers
Coming for Treatment

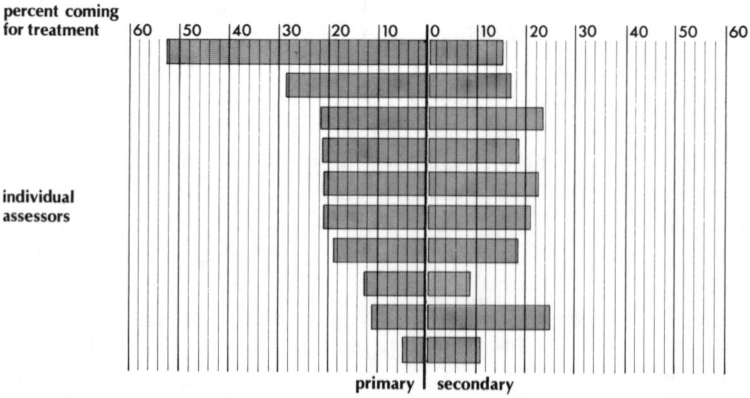

There were clear patterns of antecedent and concurrent factors leading to the social adaptational problems as well as to self-reports of psychological distress. However, none of these motivated teenagers to come in for help. These results suggest that peer leaders, who are both designated and perceived as leaders and have a still unknown personal characteristic(s), are major factors in why teenagers come for help.

Mechanic (1970) indicates that a broad array of factors influence help-seeking. Symptoms may play some but not the entire role in accounting for who goes to second-level and third-level patient status. Selective forces influence individuals to seek treatment, especially in the case of children, who are most often not in control of the choice. Social and family factors may be as important or more important in determining who appears for treatment as the nature of the disorder itself.

Further research is badly needed to understand the processes in screening and influencing people to come for help. There should be careful epidemiologic studies that examine who comes for treatment and who does not; those who receive help at the second and third levels will be compared with those in the populations who do not in terms of the severity and kinds of need they have and other potential influences. The most important point to be made here is that the patients at the second and third levels cannot be assumed to represent the ill population from the first level.

The Concept of Community

Epidemiologic research in child psychiatry is possibly most useful when done in particular kinds of communities and then replicated in the same and deliberately varied other kinds of communities. The advantage of community epidemiologic research in child psychiatry is that the concept of community focuses upon the familial, educational, political, and economic institutions, along with the physical environment, which might enhance or inhibit the mental health or illness of the child. Variation in the families, in the schools and their classrooms, and in peer groups within a particular kind of community can be studied in regard to their contribution to the child's psychiatric condition.

In 1913, Adolf Meyer wrote concerning the importance of the local community: "I consider it of the greatest importance that the clinic make itself responsible for the mental health work of a fairly well circumscribed unit of population, so as to make possible studies of the dynamic factors which lead to the occurrence of mental derangements which must be attacked for purposes of prevention" (Meyer, 1951, p. 194). He was referring to the opportunity that such a "unit of population" holds to study the kinds of circumstances over the life course of individuals which might influence their illness or health.

Defining the community and its boundaries becomes important both in allowing epidemiologic studies within a particular population and in integrating services. Integrating services may have not only utilitarian functions of treatment or prevention, but may also be important in experimentally testing theoretical ideas of causation. Major social change can also be studied in quasi experiments. If we hypothesize, for example, that the shame and stigma of being on welfare may trigger depression in susceptible individuals in some communities and not others, then the negative income tax experiments done in a specifically defined variety of communities would have theoretical as well as practical importance as a way of testing this hypothesis (Ensminger, 1978; Thoits and Hannan, 1979).

The word "community" needs to be examined, however, since from the above discussion it should be clear that community cannot be defined merely by drawing arbitrary lines around areas on a map. Such a process would not be likely to coincide with the local citizens' views or with the existing social and political structure. Roland Warren (1963) defines community as: " . . . that combination of social units and systems which perform the major social functions having locality relevance. This is another way of saying that by community we mean the organization of social activities to afford people daily local access to those broad areas of activity which are necessary in day-to-day living" (p. 10). Many neighborhoods, urban and rural, would more or less qualify as communities. Such areas are most often identified by a local name. In addition, they usually have known boundaries, their own shopping facilities, various neighborhood voluntary associations, and health and welfare services. Communities may also have locally based political organizations which play a role in city, state, and federal politics.

We should not have any romantic illusions that neighborhoods or communities provide enduring or even the most important roots for people. Americans are geographically mobile. However, communities may be important for several reasons. First, communities may serve important functions that are somewhat independent of the population that at any one time resides in them. For example, ecological studies have long shown that within urban areas there are neighborhoods that have been the entry point to the city for various ethnic groups (Shaw and McKay, 1969). As soon as the entering population has become established within the city, it moves to other, more prestigious and comfortable neighborhoods, making way for later entering groups. Or a community may serve as a "bedroom" residential area for a metropolitan area. By recognizing the function that different communities serve, the epidemiologist may focus not only on the individual characteristics of the population but also on the social structure and ecological processes going on within that community and their impact on the illness or disorder being studied.

Especially important to those interested in children is the concept of the "community of limited liability" (Janowitz, 1967; Suttles, 1972). This concept recognizes that the local community may not be very relevant for many feelings or activities of the urbanized American; however, the community may have more importance for certain groups (e.g., the very old and the very young) than others. The young are limited in their freedom of geographic mobility; the main activities of play and school usually take place within the local neighborhood. Services designed for the young such as educational, recreational, and medical services, are usually provided in local settings. For those researchers and clinicians, then, who focus on children and families, the local community may be particularly important.

Our own research illustrates how longitudinal epidemiologic studies may follow a community population even though they may be "alumni" of the community. Between 1964 and 1969 we assessed the mental health of all the first graders in Woodlawn at several points in each school year. The children were assessed again when they reached third grade. In the spring of 1965 and the spring of 1967, we conducted interviews with the mothers or mother surrogates of the children who were in first grade in those two years. These assessments were coupled with service and evaluation programs which were partly directed at systematically developing community-wide prevention and early intervention programs. In all of these service and research ventures we had the cooperation and support of a community board composed of leaders from the community's larger citizen organizations, and assistance of the board has been essential throughout the course of this work (Kellam and Branch, 1971; Kellam et al., 1972).

As part of a 10-year follow-up, in 1975–76 we reinterviewed the mothers or mother surrogates and the children from the 1966–67 first-grade classes. Though our population originally lived in Woodlawn, by the time of follow-up about 70% of these children and families lived elsewhere in the Chicago metropolitan area. About eight of every 10 of the mobile families lived in areas with better housing and higher median incomes. The epidemiologic map on the next page shows the 1975 location of those 1966–67 Woodlawn first-grade families who comprised the follow-up population. The dots are map tacks indicating their location in 1975. (The dispersion is so broad that the map seems to suggest that most families were still in Woodlawn, but in fact only about 30% still resided there in 1975.) The numbers assigned to communities are those traditionally used for Chicago neighborhood areas (see, e.g., Shaw and McKay's [1969] pioneer epidemiologic studies of delinquency and Faris and Dunham's [1939] of psychiatric illness).

The broad dispersion of the follow-up extends over the south and southwest areas of Chicago. This high rate of mobility and extensive spread was not expected by Chicago urban planners and demographers, who, like us, thought of Woodlawn as a relatively static area providing little opportunity for upward social mobility. These data require the study of the impact of geographic and social mobility and stability of residence on important adolescent psychological and social outcomes.

The map presents compelling evidence that the concept of community cannot be defined in static terms. While the child is growing and the family evolving, the community may be doing the same. Community must be thought of as having an evolving course, presenting a changing social, political, economic, and even physical environment as background for the life-span development of the child. For child psychiatric epidemiology, this means that relevant aspects of community must be measured, along with variables in the child and whatever other variables are under study, in order not to mistake change in the community for change in the child.

The Concept of the Family

In our culture there has been a general acceptance of the importance of the child-rearing family to the long-term growth and development of the child. Almost all family research has been done on the nuclear family, that is, mother, father, and children. Those investigators interested in comparing types of families have most often used dichotomies, such as intact vs. nonintact families or father-present vs. father-absent families. In an extensive summary of the father-absent literature, Herzog and Sudia (1973) concluded that the results are ambiguous and that the importance of father absence to child rearing may be mediated and/or influenced by other factors of greater importance. Most researchers specifically

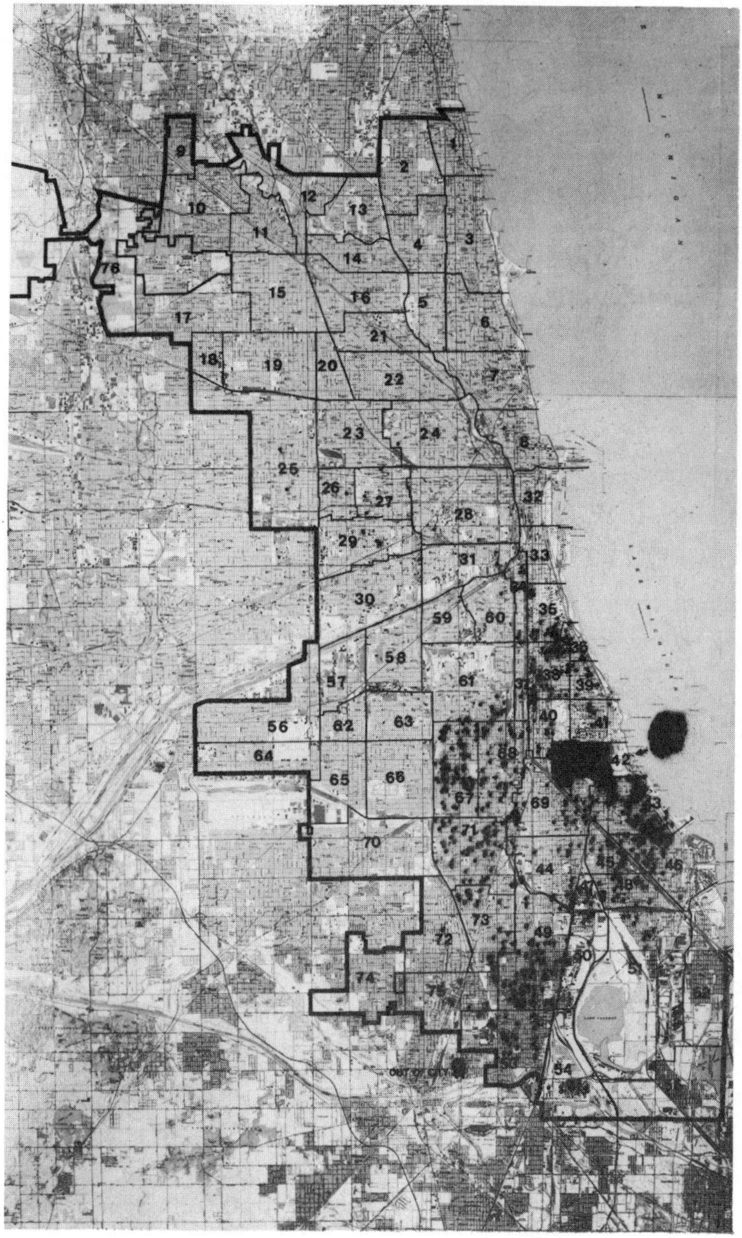
1
2
3
4
5
6
7
8
9
10
11
12
13
14
15
16
17
18
19
20
21
22
23
24
25
26
27
28
29
30
31
32
33
35
36
39
40
41
42
44
45
46
49
50
51
54
56
57
58
59
60
61
62
63
64
65
66
67
68
69
70
71
72
73
74
75
76
OUT OF CITY

interested in the development of mental health and illness also have studied the nuclear family with little attention to other types. We attribute this concentration (1) to the historical importance in our culture of the nuclear family and (2) to a strong consensus among Americans of all social classes and ethnic groups that the mother/father family is inherently superior (Schneider, 1968).

A current crucial issue in child psychiatry is the evaluation of how important the family is and what aspects of family are important to the long-term evolving mental health of the child. This perspective, of course, is a departure from the general acceptance of the power of the family on the potential of the individual. In a recent monograph Clarke and Clarke (1976) gather evidence from their own work and that of others which suggests a potential for later development beyond early child rearing. They call for review of the role of family:

> Our main general conclusion is that, in man, early learning is mainly important for its foundational character. By itself, and when repeated over time, it serves as no more than a link in the developmental chain, shaping proximate behaviour less and less powerfully as age increases . . . Our major research need in this important area is to determine more precisely the factors that initiate, accentuate and maintain alteration in human characteristics as well as to determine the ultimate limits of these effects and the causes of individual differences in responsiveness to change. (1976, p. 18).

Neugarten (1979) and Kagan (1979) argue in a similar vein for such a life-span developmental approach.

We will illustrate our concern with this issue by examining a central aspect of family structure (i.e., the different combinations of adults present in child-rearing households), its relationship to the mental health of young schoolchildren, and its evolution over a 10-year period. The study of variations in the constellation of adults present in the home is a basic aspect of family structure and is of great importance because roles in the family will depend on its composition. The addition or deletion of certain adults; the age, spacing, and number of children; marital history; and the life-cycle stages of the various members of the family may influence the nature of family roles, other aspects of family life, and the well-being of family members.

Family types at the time of first grade were classified in terms of the adults at home on the basis of information obtained in the interviews with the mothers or mother surrogates of the first-grade children (Kellam et al., 1977). A taxonomy of the various combinations of adults present in the households of the 1966–67 population of first graders is shown in fig. 2. We found 10 different adult relatives present in the families, plus four residual categories of male and female relatives and nonrelatives. There were 86 different combinations of these adults in 1966–67, while in 1964–65 there were 79 combinations.

Figure 2 is cumulative from top to bottom. If one begins, for instance, at the upper left hand corner with mother alone, and descends directly down to mother/father and then to mother/father/grandmother, it may be seen that mother-alone families occur 517 times, mother/father 483 times, mother/father/grandmother 10 times, mother/father/grandmother/aunt only once. When a combination does not contain the next relative listed in the left and right margins, it is shown by a line moving laterally and downward to the next included relative. Thus there are 38 mother/grandmother families, four mother/grandmother/aunt families; and so on.

Eight major classes of families plus a residual "other" category may be seen in the conelike clustering of family types. These are named across the bottom of the figure. These nine, plus mother-alone families, yield 10 major classes of families raising first-grade children in Woodlawn in 1966–67. The taxonomy derived from the 1964–65 first-grade families was almost identical to this one.

The taxonomy illustrates that great diversity exists in households of first-grade children in this community. We have no reason to assume that considerable variation would not be an important characteristic of other kinds of communities. Some of the family types are relatively rare and, though intriguing, are difficult to study because of infrequent occurrence (for example, the father who is raising a first grader with no other adult in the home). Categories can be collapsed for analytic purposes in ways informed by the taxonomy and by the results of other studies.

In Woodlawn, family type was found to be strongly related to the child's social adaptational status (SAS) and psychological well-being (PWB) at least as far as third grade. The results in both study populations suggest that (1) mother-alone families entail the highest risk to the SAS and PWB of the child; (2) the presence of certain second adults has important ameliorative functions—mother/grandmother families are nearly as effective as mother/father families, with mother/stepfather families similar in risk to mother alone; and (3) in terms of risk, the absence of the father was less important than the aloneness of the mother.

From the life-span developmental perspective, these studies were important because they illustrate two of the three main perspectives described by investigators in this area (Baltes et al., 1980). First, there was a clear relationship between family structure and the

FIGURE 2

VARIATION IN FAMILIES OF WOODLAWN FIRST GRADE CHILDREN (1966-1967)

1391 FAMILIES

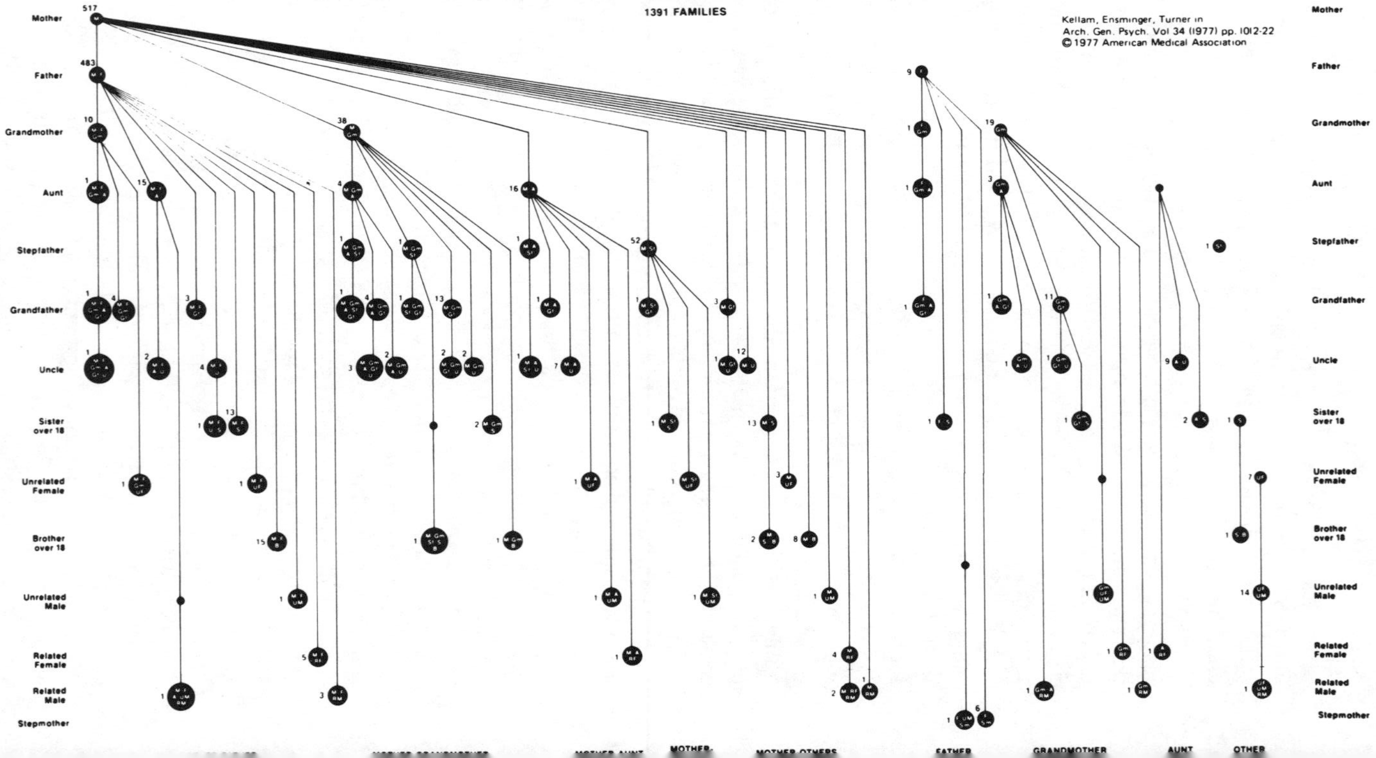

child's social adaptation to school and his or her PWB. Second, while these relationships were found in both the 1964–65 and the 1966–67 first-grade populations, there was at the same time a marked shift in the baseline percentage of maladapting children in these two separate groups. This result is a cohort effect which changed the frequencies of social maladaptation but left the relationships of family structure to social adaptation and PWB intact. Cohort effects must be taken into account as a major source of behavior determinism (Baltes et al., 1978).

We will describe some of the major impacts of teenage motherhood on family structure to illustrate further how specifying family structure may be important in child psychiatric epidemiology. In recent years many people have been concerned by what is felt to be a marked increase in teenage childbearing. This concern seems to be based on the belief, increasingly supported by evidence, that women who start childbearing early in life are at a disadvantage that makes it difficult for them to care for their children adequately. Teenage motherhood is often associated with indicators of the deterioration of the family (Trussell, 1976) such as marital instability (Norton and Glick, 1976), welfare dependency (Moore and Caldwell, 1977), and illegitimacy (Baldwin, 1976; Osofsky, 1970).

FIGURE 3

Age of Mother at Birth of Child and Family Type at First Grade

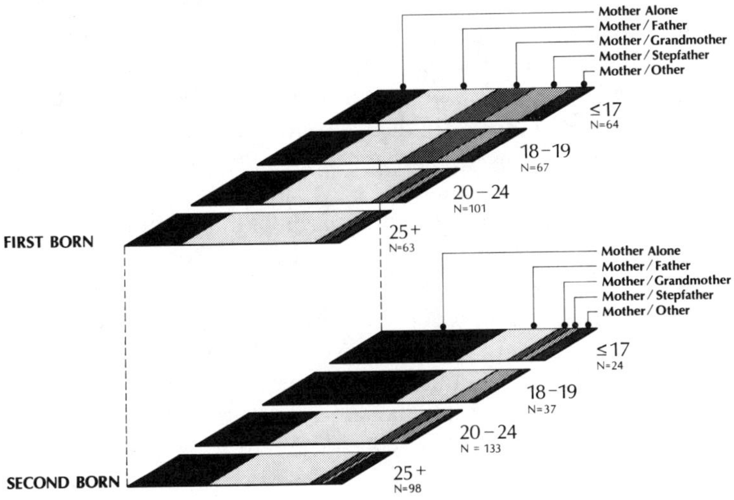

Figure 3 shows how family structure varies in Woodlawn by virtue of teenage mothering. The frequency of different kinds of family structure, indicated by the age of mother at the birth of her first child, is shown for both firstborn and second-born children. Children later than second-born have been left out in order to show the impact of mother's age on family structure within a relatively early portion of the mother's child-rearing stage (Kellam et al., 1980a).

For both firstborn and second-born children, family structure is clearly related to the mother's age at the birth of her first child (Kellam et al., 1980a). Six years after the birth of the child being studied, older mothers (those over 20) were more likely than teenage mothers to be in mother/father families. Well over half of the older mothers lived with the child's father. About one-third of the teenage mothers of firstborn children, but only one-fifth of teenage mothers of second-born children, lived with father.

A substantial number of teenage mothers with firstborn children lived in households with their own mothers, but teenage mothers with two children were much more likely to be living alone with their children. (In testing the independence of firstborn or second-born status and family type for the four age groups we have, in order of increasing age, $\chi^2 = 9.3, 10.8, 0.1, 3.8$ each on 2 df; the first two age categories—the teenage ones—are significant.) For most of our analyses we combined into one category the mothers of first-born and second-born children because it did not affect the relationships of age of mother to evolving family structure other than in the important ways just described.

The tendency of teenage mothers to either begin in or evolve toward mother-alone households with the addition of later children is further demonstrated when we examine the family structure 10 years later, at the time of long-term follow-up. Figure 4 illustrates this trend toward aloneness in the case of those mothers who were in mother/father families at first grade in 1966–67 (noted by the shaded rectangle at that point along the time axis). Each category of age of mother (defined by age at birth of first child) is shown separately. The family structures in which the mothers in a particular age category lived 10 years later are shown in the rectangle at the right side of each graphic. Those mothers we could not reinterview are also shown in this rectangle. We did not interview as many mothers who began childbearing as teenagers as we did older mothers. This was due to a higher refusal rate among mothers who began child rearing as teenagers. As we describe later, this seems to

FIGURE 4

The Evolution of Mother/Father Families by Age of Mother

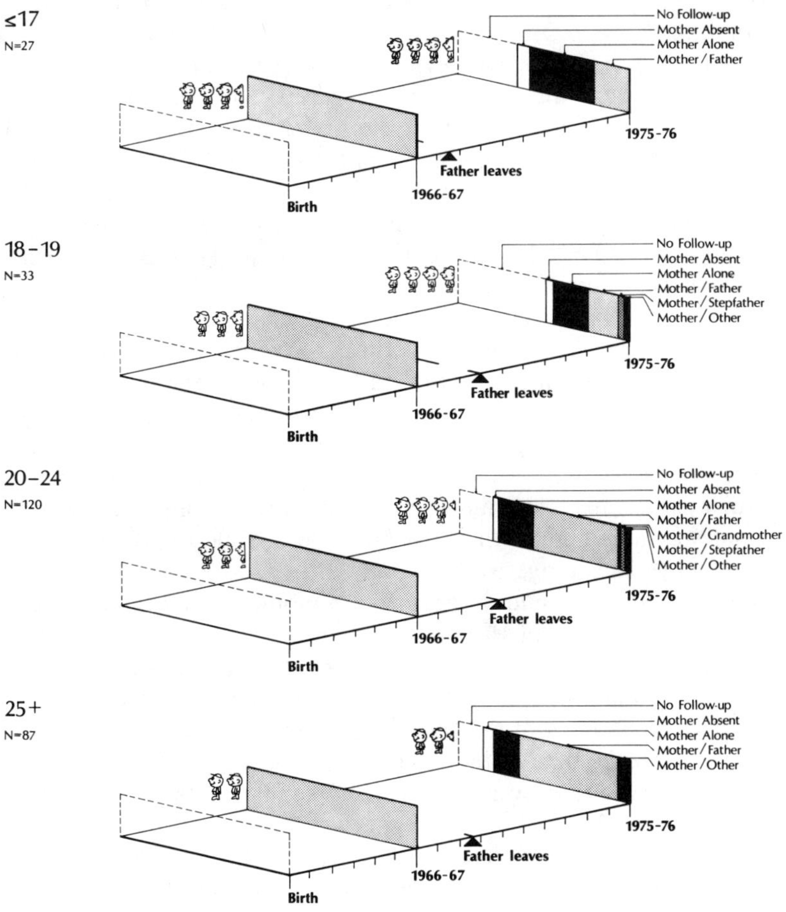

be another indication of the aloneness of teenage mothers. The average number of children at these two times are shown, as well as the mean age of the child when father left if he did leave.

Among those we reinterviewed, the stability of the mother/father family with a teenage mother was dramatically different from that of the mother/father family with an older mother. While 33% of the youngest teenagers and 38% of the older teenagers remained in mother/father families, 62% of the 20–24-year-old mothers and 68% of the mothers 25 years old or older remained in mother/father families.

A teenage mother originally in mother/father families was likely to be the only adult in the family at the time of reinterview. Mother/stepfather households were not a frequent alternative at the time of reinterview for the mothers from the 1967 mother/father families of any age group. The evolutions in structure of mother/father families for different age groups were not at all similar (χ = 13.6 on 3 df, $p < .01$) and represent important contrasts between teenage and older mothers.

In mother/father families from which the father had left, the separation occurred at different times for different age groups of mothers. (The mean age of the study child when the father left is marked along the time axis between first grade and follow-up.) Teenage mothers who were in mother/father families when their firstborn or second-born was in first grade tended to separate from father earlier than older mothers. For the latter, the mean age of the child was about nine when the father left, while for the teenage mothers the mean age was 7.6.

The number of children born to the mother/father families decreased as the age of the mother increased ($p < .01$ by F-test). (Child figures depict the average number of children.) The mothers aged 25 or older had, on the average, one less birth in the first six years after the birth of the study child than the mothers aged 17 or younger. By the time of follow-up the mothers aged 17 or younger had, on the average, over 1.5 more children than mothers aged 25 or older.

Figure 4 also shows that we successfully reinterviewed a smaller proportion of the teenage mothers than of the older mothers. This tendency was due to the refusal of teenage mothers to be reinterviewed rather than our inability to find them. Refusal to be reinterviewed was associated with a pattern of social disconnectedness.

Mothers who were the only adult in their household attended church services less and participated in church organizations and social and political organizations less than other mothers. They reported much less help in child rearing in such areas as providing opportunities for the child to confide, setting and enforcing rules, and affectional activities with the child (Kellam et al., 1980a; Brown et al., 1980, in our lab have also demonstrated a short-and long-term risk of increased psychological distress in teenage mothers.)

We have attempted to illustrate in this section the vital importance of systematic specification of family structure in child psychiatric epidemiologic research. Here we have noted that, for children of mother-alone families, both early social adaptation and PWB are at high risk at this time and in this kind of community; that the families of teenage mothers, as an example of an important variable in influencing family structure, strongly tend to evolve toward mother-alone households; and that the long-term evolution of mother-alone families is associated with a disconnectedness in social organizational membership and help in child rearing.

Specification of core characteristics of family is vitally important in child psychiatric research, in the context of defined characteristics of the community. Since studies of total populations are necessary in order to determine the frequencies and consequences of various kinds of family structure that occur in a particular population, this specification can best be done through epidemiologic research.

A life-span developmental perspective has been either explicit or implicit in much of the preceding discussion. Baltes et al. (1980) recently summarized this theoretical orientation with examples in empirical research. The main contribution stems from the focus on the three main sources of determinism of behavior over the life course. The first, normative/ontogenetic, is concerned with developmental and socialization influences. A second, normative/historical, refers to cohort effects, or the evolving history or background of the community, society, or culture in which the individual is developing and being socialized. In other words, while early developmental and socialization processes lead to later behavior, there is also an evolving societal history which is unfolding and influencing these processes and the behavioral outcomes of the individual. A third, nonnormative source is that of idiosyncratic life events which befall an individual and which may not be typical of other individuals in the particular population. Stressful life events represent a simple view of this source of determinism of later behavior.

Child psychiatric epidemiologic research must keep in view these three potential sources of determinism. While all research investigations may not be able to measure all three sources, they must nonetheless be considered in the strength and kind of inferences to be drawn from research.

Social Adaptational Status and Psychological Well-Being: A Two-Dimensional View of Mental Health and Illness

A major problem in relating theory and method in child psychiatric epidemiology is the lack of a coherent conceptual framework for defining disorders for children (Achenbach, 1978) in spite of the very informative reliability studies that compared the DSM-II and DSM-III in the diagnosis of childhood and adolescent psychiatric disorders (Cantwell et al., 1979a, 1979b; Mattison et al., 1979; Russell et al., 1979). We lack evidence for the validity of many child diagnostic categories in DSM-III and the other nosological systems. This is particularly true for conduct problems and other areas where social behavior is central. The fact that a person comes to a clinic is often assumed to reflect psychiatric disorder. In epidemiologic research, the clinic cannot be assumed to be a screener of health/illness; and we have described the factors that influence seeking help at second and third level agencies. The total population of children must be examined for specific, systematically defined indices of illness or disorder.

One of the most striking differences between assessments made in the clinic and those made in epidemiologic sites is that social role performance and its relation to psychiatric disorder become more prominent in the epidemiologic site. The classroom, for example, is often the epidemiologic locus of observing and rating children for child psychiatric disorder. In the process, one sees children who, in the view of the teacher, are misbehaving, others who are behaving similarly but with the teacher's approval, still others who are misbehaving and appear anxious, others who are misbehaving but appear psychologically comfortable, and so on.

In the Woodlawn studies, we have considered it important to distinguish between social role performance and psychological status. While the two may be empirically related (and in the Woodlawn research we found this to be the case), they are nevertheless conceptually quite different, and the relationships we have found are by no means simple. Many more first grade children were thought by their teachers to be maladapting than were symptomatic in the view of observing clinicians. The short- and long-term courses of social role performance and psychological well-being were strikingly different and their interrelationships very specific. Other investigators (Robins, 1966; Robins, 1978; Watt, 1978; Loney, 1980) have reported similar findings.

In considering this two-dimensional view, and in particular the role performance aspect, the following conceptual framework may help. We have called it the Life Course-Social Field Concept (Kellam et al., 1975). It is based on the theoretical development of Erikson (1959, 1963), Havighurst (1952), Neugarten (1968), and others over the last several decades.

Every individual in society passes through stages of life, which at certain times seem more clear and at others more vague (Neugarten, 1979). Each stage involves that individual in specific social fields in which there are persons who define social tasks and judge the adequacy of the individual's performance in that field. Such persons, whom we have termed "natural raters" (NR in the figure), are similar to Lippitts's "socialization agents" (1968).

The parents at home, the teacher in the classroom, the foreman at work are examples of such persons in specific social fields. The process involved is highly interactional, and we have named it "social adaptation." The natural raters rate the adequacy of each individual's performance, sometimes very formally as teachers do with grades, sometimes informally as in parental attitudes about how well the child is behaving. We conceive of this interactional process as the basic interface between the individual and society.

Social adaptational status—the adequacy of performance as rated by the natural rater in a specific social field—is a societal judgment of the individual's performance and is therefore external to the individual. Stages of life as defined by Havighurst (1952) are shown in fig. 5 combined with a series of major life events, which often occur at times of transition from one stage to the next. This chart demonstrates how the stages of life and the major life events intersect with specific social fields, such as the family, the classroom, or work.

The figure presents a generalized interpretation of the individual's life course. For many individuals in Woodlawn and in different communities or societies, variations from this idealized pattern will be frequent (Neugarten, 1979).

Variations in the width of the horizontal bars representing each social field are intended to suggest the relative importance of each field at different stages, and this, too, will vary among individuals, communities, and societies. Everyone is not involved in rearing young children in early adulthood, nor does every adult function in the work context. Still, the concept is useful in that it illustrates the relationship between an individual's stage of life and important aspects of societal structure and function.

In contradistinction to SAS, there is the question of how the individual is feeling inside, that is, his or her PWB. By PWB we mean the thought processes, affective status, self-esteem, and other aspects of the psychological status of the individual.

These two components—SAS and PWB—represent the two major dimensions of mental health. One represents mental health from the viewpoint of society; the other represents mental health from the viewpoint of the individual. This two-dimensional concept of mental health builds on a variety of concepts from social and behavioral sciences. Charles Horton Cooley and George Herbert Mead were both concerned with the individual's perception of how others see him and its effect on his sense of self (Cooley, 1922; Mead, 1934).

From an epidemiologic standpoint, the social fields represent the locations within the community where the individuals at a particular stage of life can be found. Equally important, within each social field can also be found the natural rater. In defining social tasks and rating the individuals within the social fields, the natural raters are the sources of social adaptational measures for the epidemiologic investigator. For child psychiatric epidemiology, the family and the classroom are the two major social fields in which young children can be found, and parents in the home and teachers in the classroom are the natural raters. Very soon the peer group becomes a major locus also. In the Woodlawn epidemiologic studies, we assumed that the peer group in first grade was not yet a major social field. Young children did not seem to influence each other and show friendship preferences with the same degree of structure and stability as later, in second grade and upward.

Chance and idiosyncracy may play a large role in SAS. Indirect measures, of course, can be made by reports from those in a position to know what the natural rater's ratings are. The validity of the indirect SAS measures may be a problem, however. Reliability of SAS measures is usually the test-retest variety, rather than interrater agreement, because there often is only one teacher in a classroom or only one foreman at the job. In most social fields such natural raters carry sole authority, and another person's opinion, no matter how expert, often does not carry the authority of the natural rater.

Adequacy of role performance as discussed by Parsons (1964) was one of the sources of our concept of SAS:

> The primary criteria for mental illness must be defined with reference to the social role-performance of the individual. Since it is at the level of role structure that the principal direct interpenetration of social systems and personalities comes to focus, it is as an incapacity to meet the expectations of social roles that mental illness becomes a problem in social relationships, and that criteria of its presence or absence should be formulated. This is of course not at all to say that the state which we refer to as mental, as opposed to somatic, illness is not a state of the individual; of course it is. But that state is manifest to and presents problems for both the sick person and others with whom he associates in the context of social relationships, and it is with reference to this problem that we are making the point about role-performance. (P. 258)

FIGURE 5

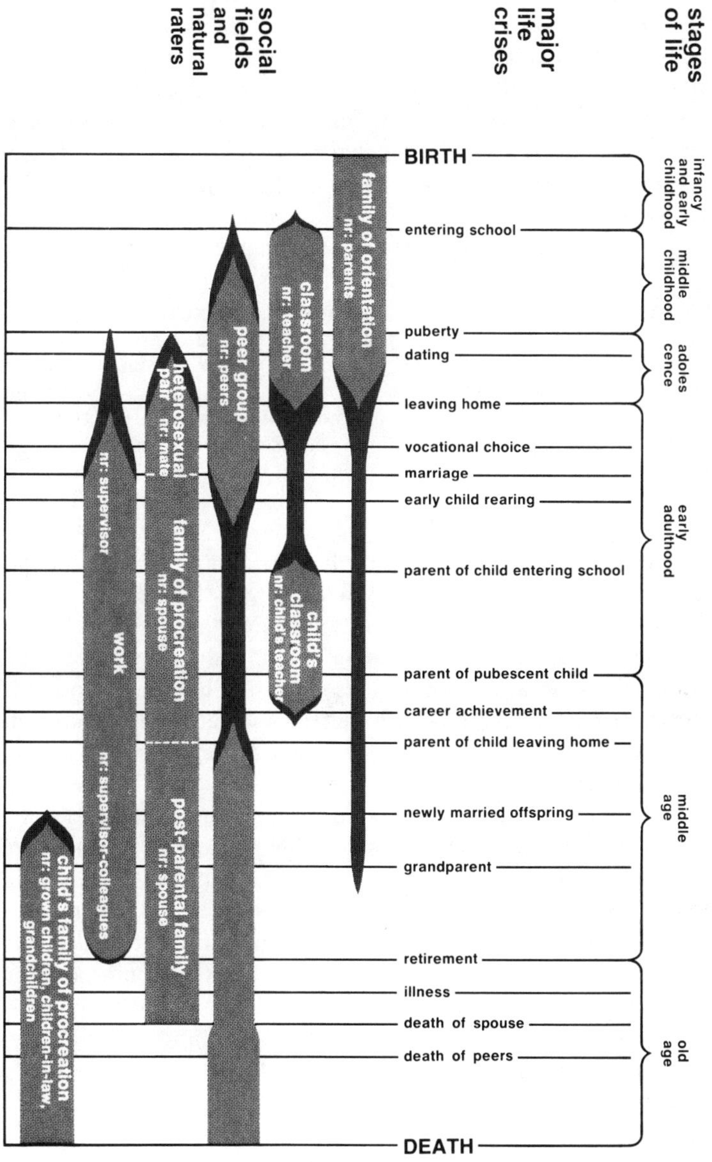

LIFE COURSE—SOCIAL FIELD CONCEPT

Social adaptational status is an elaboration of Parsons's role theory in that SAS further specifies the relationship between stages of life and specific social fields and the manner in which social tasks are presented to the individual by specific person(s) in each social field, who have societal authority to define the tasks and rate the individual's performance. The social adaptational process and the resultant SAS of an individual occur in a social field, which is part of the social structure and function of the broader society. The larger society has impact on the characteristics of each social field, and therefore on the social tasks presented the individual and on his or her SAS—an idea which reminds us of Merton's thoughts regarding the influence of the broader society on the individual:

> Our primary aim is to discover how some social structures exert a definite pressure upon certain persons in the society to engage in non-conforming rather than conforming conduct. If we can locate groups peculiarly subject to such pressures, we should expect to find fairly high rates of deviant behavior, not because the human beings comprising them are compounded of distinctive biological tendencies, but because they are responding normally to the social situation in which they find themselves. (Merton, 1968, p. 186)

We would further add that not all individuals under particular social circumstances behave in a nonconforming fashion. Nor is the response of an individual to certain social circumstances only to be found in behavior rather than also in that individual's psychological status. Such elaboration necessitates including biological and psychological perspectives along with Merton's social structural considerations in attempting to specify causes of disorder or illness and even growth and development.

Measures of SAS can be obtained by first systematically asking the natural raters in a specific social field what social tasks are expected. Then scales can be made and the natural raters asked in standardized fashion to rate the children in their social field regarding each child's performance on each task. This procedure was followed in Woodlawn with the teachers in the classrooms and the mothers at home.

In contrast to SAS, PWB is an internal state, and measures can only be inferred from self-reports of individuals, particularly as the child grows older and becomes more competent to report; from reports of significant others such as parents, teachers, or peers; and/or observations of clinicians, who use reports of others as well as direct observation of the children.

Mental health clinicians and research investigators have most often viewed these two perspectives, SAS and PWB, as opposite sides of the same coin. Psychological status is usually considered primary, with social maladaptation the measure of illness and its severity. Educators, including classroom teachers of young children, have tended to do the opposite, viewing the social adaptation of the child as primary and the psychological status or presence of psychological symptoms as a measure of severity. They too assume that these two perspectives are opposite sides of the same coin, but a different coin than that seen by the mental health professional.

By recognizing the conceptual distinctness of SAS on one hand and PWB on the other, we clarify at least one of the core problems mental health investigators have confronted for many years over the definition of mental health and illness. The SAS measure is based on coding social tasks required by natural raters and obtaining assessments by the natural raters of the performance of the child. In contrast, PWB measures are obtained by coding the dimensions of PWB that are of interest and obtaining inferred measures of the various internal dimensions of the child's psychic life.

By separating these two dimensions, we are able to investigate their interrelation over time and to discover the long-term outcomes of each. Such investigation has been at the center of attention in the Woodlawn studies, and the results suggest that SAS in first grade in particular has very important long-term predictive and possibly developmental significance at least as far as adolescence. These results tend to be similar to those found by Robins (1966), for example, in her studies of the long-term importance of early aggressiveness to adult clinic and criminal outcome. Watt (1978) also has recently reported the long-term importance of aggressiveness in young males as an antecedent of schizophrenia in adulthood. Loney (1980) has shown evidence that early aggressiveness is the key prognostic component of the hyperactivity syndrome. While there are modest correlations in longitudinal studies between early PWB and later PWB or SAS, the evidence from our research and other studies suggests that the psychological dimension does not have the same importance to long-term outcomes as does SAS. The circumstances which influence these long-term relationships of SAS to PWB and the relationships of each to other outcomes requires much more prospective longitudinal, community epidemiologic research.

The adequacy of social role performance is a societal judgment. As child psychiatric investigators we must accept it as a part of the reality in the child's world. Our job is to investigate its causes, not merely to assume that social maladaptation is only a reflection of the child's psychological status. The locus of problems such as "hyperactivity" cannot be assumed to be in the child, although it may be in some children. It must be part of our measurement of mental health and illness to find out. We can only do so if we separate SAS from PWB and measure each in a manner that enables us to study their interrelationships over time.

Investigators into psychopathology have frequently complained about this position, since they often feel there is no alternative to using SAS as a criterion of illness. We suggest that the solution is to measure symptoms and other aspects of psychological status, to measure SAS independently, and to empirically study their interrelationships over time. Such a strategy can be done in conjunction with measures of the diagnostic categories, to allow research into their validity.

The concept of diagnostic categories is an old one in medicine. Its application to psychiatry has been accepted with great enthusiasm at certain times and rejected at others. Criteria vary from one period to another. Recently, new methods intended to increase reliability and validity have been developed. Diagnostic criteria have been incorporated and reliability in many categories improved (Spitzer et al., 1980). At the least, greater uniformity in our diagnostic language has been achieved.

The validity of many diagnostic categories requires much more study, however (see Kendell, 1979; Carpenter et al., 1980; Kendell et al., 1980; Gift et al., 1980; Loney, 1980; Shaffer, 1979). Such research requires measuring symptoms separately from each other and from SAS. Only by longitudinal epidemiologic study of these separate areas can we determine whether the components of a diagnostic category actually have a common or developmental course together.

Child psychiatric epidemiology particularly requires such a strategy since there is even less evidence at the early stage of life of continuity of psychological measures with adult psychopathology. This is not to say that continuities do not exist, but our determination of what they are is not yet sufficient to measure only diagnostic categories rather than the components of PWB and SAS separately, along with the diagnostic categories.

Biological, psychological, and social determinants of health and illness hypothetically may operate at any level of organization: (1) at the level of general distress; (2) at the level of specific symptoms; and/or (3) at the level of specific diagnostic categories (Buchsbaum and Rieder, 1979). Weissman et al. (1979) have recently done a very important kind of study examining the longitudinal relationship of self-reports of depressive symptoms to depressive illness. Such epidemiologic studies will provide greater understanding of the relationships among the above defined three levels of organization of psychopathology and the validity of each.

Biological, social, and psychological determinants could also operate on PWB or on SAS or both. Child psychiatric epidemiology requires data, therefore, on illness or disorder measured at all three levels of organization of psychological distress, and with PWB and SAS also measured separately.

Illustrations from Longitudinal Analyses on Woodlawn Data—We have defined SAS and PWB as separate concepts in the Woodlawn studies, and have measured them independently of each other, so that we might study their long-term interrelationships and the outcome of each. We will illustrate with analyses of the antecedents of teenage drug use, a social behavioral outcome, comparing these results with the antecedents of self-reports of psychological distress, an internal psychological outcome.

In order to obtain SAS measures in first grade, we obtained from the 57 first grade teachers in 12 elementary schools in Woodlawn lists of tasks which they expected first grade children to perform (see Kellam et al., 1975). We then inferred five main social tasks suggested by these: (1) socializing with other children, speaking up, and not sitting alone too much; (2) obeying rules and not fighting; (3) demonstrating sufficient independence so as not to be too clinging to the teacher; (4) learning up to ability as the teacher sees it; and (5) paying attention and being able to concentrate on tasks. Global scales were constructed on the basis of these tasks and standardized interviews were carried out with each of the first grade teachers at three points in first grade and again in third grade, on four consecutive cohorts of total first grade population.

Children whose teachers rated them maladapting on any one scale of SAS most often were rated maladapting on other scales as well. We have studied the scales as well as typal categories, and generally have found that typal categories based on the presence or absence of shyness, aggressiveness, and learning problems, are most useful in describing a child's pattern of social maladaptation. Shyness and aggressiveness are described above. Learning problems consisted of maladapting on any or all of the other three scales: being sufficiently independent or unclinging; learning up to the teacher's perception of the child's ability; and paying attention. (Kohn and Rossman [1972] and Lambert and Nicholl [1977] developed similar typologies.) Shyness, aggressiveness, and learning problems are three kinds of social maladaptation and are distinct from symptoms of anxiety or depression, which are internal feelings rather than maladapting at social tasks.

Eight typal categories of SAS were thus derived: adapting within minimal limits; learning problems without shyness or aggressiveness; mildly shy, usually with learning problems; mildly aggressive, usually with learning problems; moderately or severely shy, almost always with learning problems; moderately or severely aggressive, almost always with learning problems; and moderately or severely shy and aggressive, almost always with learning problems. The combinations of shy and aggressive consisted of children who sat alone and had few friends and also got into fights and broke rules.

At the time of the 10-year follow-up of the 1966–67 Woodlawn first graders and their families, the study population was 16–17 years old. They provided us with self-reports of psychiatric symptoms, self-esteem, their perceptions of their own SAS in school, with family, peers, and the opposite sex, along with their satisfaction with their SAS in each of these domains. We reinterviewed the mothers along the same dimensions as in first grade, using as many identical questions as possible. In addition, information regarding drugs, alcohol, and cigarette use was obtained from both mothers and teenagers. We also collected school records, including achievement and attendance.

In the first stage of the 10-year follow-up we located and reinterviewed 939 (75%) of the mothers or mother surrogates of the 1,242 families in the 1966–67 study. Following the reinterviews of the 939 mothers, and with their permission, 705 teenagers (75%) finally participated in the reassessments. We compared the early information on the mothers that we reinterviewed with the mothers we did not. The mothers whom we could not reinterview were somewhat younger as we noted before; more mobile before and during the child's first-grade year; and their children were somewhat more likely to have been in parochial schools in first grade. We found no differences between the mothers' 1966–67 PWB, early family income, welfare status, or the variety of combinations of adults at home. We found little or no differences in the children's SAS or PWB. (For description of methods of relocation, see Agrawal et al., 1978.)

Examining possible bias in sample loss continues to be an important part of each analysis we carry out. In the case of the teenage mother studies, learning the kind of loss contributed to theory-building, as well as providing an important guide to how confident we can be in the results. Possible cohort effects are also a continuing part of analytic thinking, particularly in the long-term analyses where only one cohort was studied.

FIGURE 6

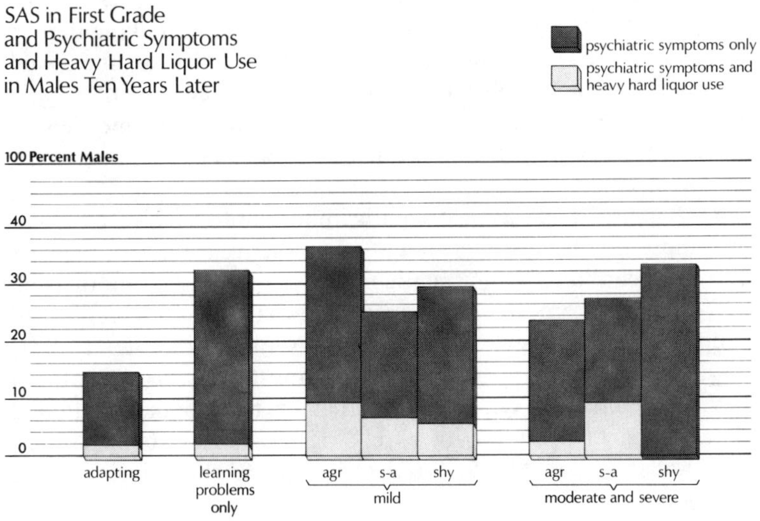

In the case of males, having learning problems in first grade, with or without shyness or aggressiveness, was associated with greater risk of psychiatric symptoms 10 years later, compared to those first-grade male children who did not. Figure 6 shows that the percentage of children who were symptomatic as teenagers is a function of their first-grade SAS ratings. While 14% of male first graders who were adapting reported high levels of psychiatric symptoms 10 years later (beyond one-half standard deviation above the mean compared to their peers) roughly 30% of male first graders who experienced learning problems with or without shyness or aggressiveness reported levels of distress beyond their peers. This total symptom score is based on Rasch model scaling, of self-reports of items of distress in the How I Feel instrument, which we have reported on elsewhere (Wright, 1977; Petersen and Kellam, 1977).

The relationship of success or failure in first grade (SAS) to male psychiatric symptoms 10 years later did not become clear early in first grade, but only became manifest by the end of first grade.

In contrast to the males, the PWB of teenage females had no relationship to early SAS. We found relations, however, between early and continuing family atmosphere and the symptom status of teenage females, but not males. Mothers' expectations of how far daughters would go in school and mothers' PWB played a role in their daughters' PWB. Teenage daughters of mothers who had had low academic expectations for the daughters in both first grade and 1975 reported more severe psychiatric symptoms than daughters of mothers who had had high expectations both times. Mothers who reported their own PWB to be poor in 1975 had daughters who reported higher symptom levels than daughters with mothers of consistently good PWB in both first grade and 1975 (Kellam et al., 1980d).

PWB in first grade seemed slightly important to females' psychiatric symptoms 10 years later, not at all predictive for males. Females who had been rated symptomatic in first grade (by their mothers on a 38-item symptom inventory) had somewhat higher self-reports of symptoms as teenagers 10 years later. Neither males nor females rated symptomatic by pairs of clinicians (using a standardized method of observing symptomatic behavior) had a higher likelihood of reporting higher levels of psychological distress 10 years later. (See Kellam et al. [1975] for descriptions of this clinical rating method.)

In regard to drug use, shy first graders used them dramatically less often 10 years later than all other teenagers in our study. Figure 7 contains data showing how male first graders within each of the first-grade SAS categories reported drug, alcohol, and cigarette use at age 16–17. The black, bottom portion of each bar represents lifetime use 20 times or more; the top, never use; and the middle portion of each bar represents 1-19 times.

Not only were the shy children infrequent drug users compared to the aggressive children, but adapting first-grade children and those with learning problems only were generally moderate drug users as teenagers. Aggressive and shy aggressive first graders were the heaviest drug users 10 years later. This relationship of shyness/aggressiveness in first grade to drug use at age 16–17 held across all of the drugs most frequently used in this community—marijuana or hashish, beer or wine, hard liquor, and cigarettes.

The above results were clearer for males than for females, although when we found the pattern for males we could discern a similar, though weaker, pattern for females.

Other early factors also influenced later drug use. Females used drugs less than males in all categories except cigarettes, where they were equal. For both males and females, higher scores on first-grade IQ and readiness-for-school tests were associated with more drug use 10 years later. These results are all main effects, showing no

FIGURE 7

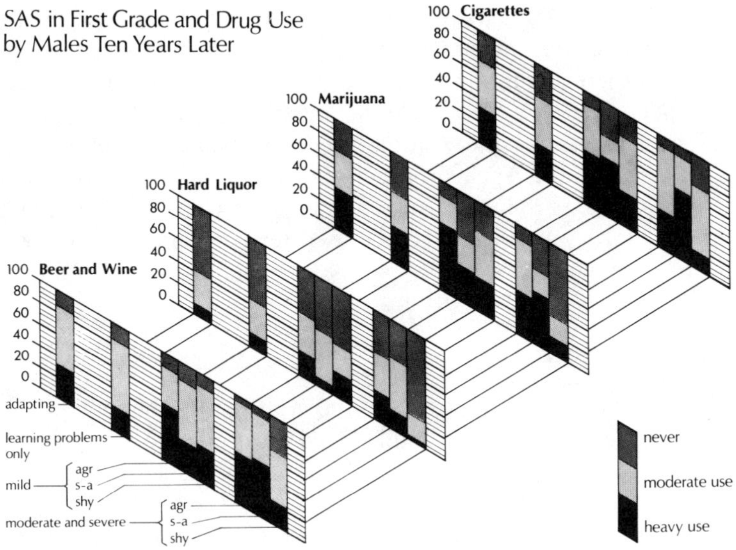

interaction among the first-grade predictors (Kellam et al., 1980c, 1980d).

A fundamental question is whether the teenagers who follow the evolutionary path to drug use are the same as those who follow the path to teenage psychiatric symptoms. Looking back now at the bar graph illustrating the relation of first-grade SAS to teenage psychiatric symptoms, we can notice the light portion at the bottom of most of the bars. This portion of the bar represents the first-grade SAS population represented by that particular bar who are both symptomatic and heavier hard liquor users 10 years later. The graph illustrates that there is little overlap in the population of those first graders who became symptomatic with the first-grade population who are also heavy hard liquor users. For example, of the moderately to severely aggressive male first graders, only 2% were both symptomatic and heavy hard liquor users 10 years later. None of the moderately or severely shy male first graders were both symptomatic and heavy hard liquor users 10 years later.

We began this chapter with a description of the functions epidemiology might play in child psychiatry. A set of problems were outlined. The solution, in our view, is to clarify and specify core theoretical constructs which would allow theory from a variety of orientations to be defined and tested. Child psychiatric epidemiologic data from Woodlawn suggest that in such communities, by the end of first grade, meaningful information can be derived which relates to the evolving life course of the child. Armed with better constructs and data, it should be possible ultimately to design prevention and early intervention programs at the community level. Equally important, such programs can be evaluated by repeated measures, leading to modification and improvement. The outpatient and hospital levels can thereby be used for more precise diagnosis and treatment.

Acknowledgements

The authors wish to acknowledge the crucial contributions of the Woodlawn community, its families and children, and the community board members who over the last 17 years have provided support and guidance for this research and service enterprise. The faculty and staffs of the Woodlawn public and Catholic elementary schools and those of the Chicago Public High Schools made crucial contributions. Over the years Dr. Curtis Melnick, former Associate Superintendent of the Chicago Board of Education, was very important to this project. Jeannette Branch, the former Director of the Woodlawn Mental Health Center and later during the follow-up the South Side Youth Program, has been involved in all aspects of the research and was responsible for the collection of the teacher ratings of social adaptational status. Mrs. Rose Bates has been an important instructor regarding community issues.

We are grateful for the assistance of our colleagues, past and present, at the Social Psychiatry Study Center in many aspects of the study. Ewalt Horwath, M.D. has made particularly important contributions on the early manuscripts of this chapter. We have cited results from studies we have co-authored with C. Hendricks Brown and Rebecca Adams. We acknowledge their contribution.

These studies have been supported by the following grants: State of Illinois Department of Mental Health Grant Numbers 17-224 and 17-322; P.H.S. Grant Number MH-15760 and Research Scientist Development Award Grant Number 1 K01-MH-47596; the Maurice Falk Medical Fund; for the critical support for the follow-up, National Institute on Drug Abuse Grant Number DA-00787, and National Institute for Child Health and Human Development Contract Number N01-H0-72871.

References

Achenbach, T.M. Psychopathology of childhood: research problems and issues. *Journal of Consulting and Clinical Psychology* 1978, *46*:759–776.

Agrawal, K.C., Kellam, S.G., Klein, Z.E., and Turner J. The Woodlawn mental health studies: tracking children and families for long-term follow-up. *American Journal of Public Health* 1978, *68*:139–142.

Baldwin, W.H. Adolescent Pregnancy and Childbearing—Growing Concerns for Americans. Washington, D.C.: Population Reference Bureau, Inc. 1980. [Mimeo addendum to Baldwin 1976, same title, *Population Bulletin 31*:3–33.]

Baltes, P.B., Cornelius, S.W., and Nesselroade, J.R. Cohort effects in behavioral development: theoretical and methodological perspectives. In *Minnesota Symposium on Child Psychology, Vol. 11,* W. A. Collins (ed.). pp. 1–63. New York: T.R. Crowell, 1978.

Baltes, P.B., Reese, H., and Lipsitt, L. Life-span developmental psychology. *Annual Review of Psychology* 1980, *31*:65–110.

Brown C.H., Adams, R.G., Kellam, S.G. A longitudinal study of teenage motherhood and symptoms of distress. To be published in *Research in Community and Mental Health, Vol. II,* R.G. Simmons (ed.). Greenwich, Connecticut: JAI Press, 1980 in press.

Buchsbaum, M.S., Rieder, R.O. Biologic heterogeneity and psychiatric research. *Archives of General Psychiatry* 1979, *36*:1163–1172.

Cantwell, D. P., Mattison, R., Russell, A.T., and Will, L. A comparison of DSM-II and DSM-III in the diagnosis of childhood psychiatric disorders, IV: Difficulties in use, global comparison, and conclusions. *Archives of General Psychiatry* 1979a., *36*:1227–1232.

Cantwell, D.P., Russell, A.T., Mattison, R., and Will, L. A comparison of DSM-II and DSM-III in the diagnosis of childhood psychiatric disorders, I: Agreement with expected diagnosis. *Archives of General Psychiatry* 1979b., *36*:1208–1216.

Carpenter, W.T., Strauss, J.S., and Bartko, J.J. Diagnostic systems and prognostic validity. Letter. *Archives of General Psychiatry* 1980, *37*:277.

Clarke, A.M., and Clarke, A.D.B., eds. *Early Experience: Myth and Evidence.* New York: The Free Press, 1976.

Cooley, C.H. *Human Nature and the Social Order.* New York: Schocken Books, 1922.

Ensminger, M.E. Welfare: social and psychological differences between recipients and non-recipients. A dissertation submitted to the faculty of the Division of the Social Sciences in candidacy for the degree of Doctor of Philosophy, Department of Sociology, University of Chicago, Chicago, Illinois. 1978.

Erikson, E.H. Identity and the life cycle, selected papers. In *Psychological Issues,* A.S. Klein (ed.). New York: International Universities Press, 1959.

Erikson, E.H.*Childhood and Society,* (rev. ed.) New York: Norton, 1963.

Faris, R.E., and Dunham, W.H. *Mental Disorders in Urban Areas.* Chicago: University of Chicago Press, 1939.

Gift, T.E., Strauss, J.S., Ritzler, B.A., Kokes, R.F., and Harder, D.W. How diagnostic concepts of schizophrenia differ. *Journal of Nervous and Mental Disease* 1980, *168*:3–8.

Havighurst, R.J. *Developmental Tasks and Education,* (2d ed.) New York: Longmans Green, 1952.

Herzog, E., and Sudia, C.E. Children in fatherless families. In *Review of Child Development Research, Vol. 3,* B.M. Caldwell and H.N. Riccuit, (eds.). Chicago: The University of Chicago Press, 1973.

Janowitz, M. *The Community Press in an Urban Setting: The Social Elements of Urbanism,* (2nd ed.). Chicago: The University of Chicago Press, 1967.

Kagan, J. The form of early development. *Archives of General Psychiatry* 1979 *36*:1047–1054.

Kellam, S.G., Adams, R.G., Brown, C.H., and Ensminger, M.E. The long-term evolution of the family structure of teenage and older mothers. Unpublished manuscript, 1980a.

Kellam, S.G., and Branch, J.D. An approach to community mental health: analysis of basic problems. *Seminars in Psychiatry 1971, 3*:207–225.

Kellam, S.G., Branch, J.D., Agrawal, K.C., and Ensminger, M.E. *Mental Health and Going to School: The Woodlawn Program of Assessment, Early Intervention and Evaluation.* Chicago: University of Chicago Press, 1975.

Kellam, S.G., Branch, J.D., Agrawal, K.C., and Grabill, M.E. Strategies in urban mental health. In *Handbook of Community Mental Health,* S.E. Golann and C. Eisdorfer, (eds.). pp. 711–727. New York: Appleton-Century-Crofts, 1972.

Kellam, S.G., Branch, J.D., Brown, C.H., and Russell, G. Why teenagers come for treatment: a ten-year prospective study of Woodlawn. *Journal of the American Academy of Child Psychiatry.* 1980b, in press.

Kellam, S.G., Ensminger, M.E., and Simon, M.B. Mental health in first grade and teenage drug, alcohol, and cigarette use. *Drug and Alcohol Dependence.* 1980c, 273–304.

Kellam, S.G., Ensminger, M.E., and Turner, R.J. Family structure and the mental health of children: concurrent and longitudinal community-wide studies. *Archives of General Psychiatry* 1977, *34*:1012–1022.

Kellam, S.G., Simon, M.B., and Ensminger, M.E. Antecedents in the first grade of teenage drug use and psychological well-being: a ten-year community-wide prospective study. In: *Prevention of Drug Abuse: Hearings Before the Select Committee on Narcotics Abuse and Control, House of Representatives, Ninety-Fifth Congress, Second Session, April 18, 20, 25, May 16, 25, 1978.* Washington, U.S. Printing Office: SCNAC-95-2-4. 1980d.

Kendell, R.E., Brockington, I.F., and Leff, J.P. Diagnostic systems and prognostic validity. Reply to Carpenter et al. *Archives of General Psychiatry* 1980, *37*:227–980

Kendell, R.E. Prognostic implications of six alternative definitions of schizophrenia. *Archives of General Psychiatry* 1979, *36*:25–31.

Kohn, M., and Rossman, B.L. A social competence scale and symptom checklist for the preschool child: factor dimensions, their cross-instrument generality, and longitudinal persistence. *Developmental Psychology* 1972, *6*:430–444.

Lambert, N., and Nicholl, R.L. A conceptual model for nonintellectual behavior and its relationship to early reading achievement. *Journal of Educational Psychology* 1977, *69*:481–490.

Lippitts, R. Improving the socialization process. In *Socialization and Society.* J.A. Clausen, (ed.). Boston: Little, Brown, 1968.

Loney, J. Hyperkinesis comes of age. What do we know and where should we go? *American Journal of Orthopsychiatry* 1980 *50*:28–42.

Mattison, R., Cantwell, D.P., Russell, A.T., and Will, L. A comparison of DSM-II and DSM-III in the diagnosis of childhood psychiatric disorders, II: Interrater agreement. *Archives of General Psychiatry* 1979, *36*:1217–1222.

Mead, G.H. *Mind, Self and Society.* Chicago: The University of Chicago Press, 1934.

Mechanic, D. Problems and prospects in psychiatric epidemiology. In *Psychiatric Epidemiology: Proceedings of the International Symposium held at Aberdeen University, 22-5 July 1969,* E.H. Hare, and J.K. Wing, (eds.). New York: Oxford University Press, 1970.

Merton, R.K. *Social Theory and Social Structure,* (rev. ed.). New York: Free Press of Glencoe, 1968.

Meyer, A. *The Collected Papers of Adolph Meyer, vol. II.* E. Winters, ed. Baltimore: The John Hopkins Press, 1951.

Moore, K., and Caldwell, S. *Out of Wedlock Childbearing.* Washington, D.C.: The Urban Institute, 1977.

Neugarten, B.L. The awareness of middle age. In *Middle Age and Aging: A Reader in Social Psychology,* B.L. Neugarten (ed.), Chicago: The University of Chicago Press, 1968.

Neugarten, B.L. Time, age, and the life cycle. *American Journal of Psychiatry* 1979, *136*:887–894.

Norton, A.J. and Glick P. Marital instability: past, present, and future. *Journal of Social Issues* 1976, *32*:5–20.

Osofsky, H.J. Teenage out-of wedlock pregnancy: some preventive considerations. *Adolescence* 1970, *5*:151–170.

Parsons, T. *Social Structure and Personality.* New York: Free Press, 1964.

Petersen, A.C., and Kellam, S.G. Measurement of the psychological well-being of adolescents: the psychometric properties and assessment procedure of the *How I Feel. Journal of Youth and Adolescence* 1977, *6*:229–247.

Robins, L.N. *Deviant Children Grown Up: A Sociological and Psychiatric Study of Sociopathic Personality.* Baltimore: Williams and Wilkins, 1966.

Robins, L.N., Sturdy childhood predictors of adult outcomes: replications from longitudinal studies. Presented at Paul Hoch Award Lecture, American Psychopathological Association Meeting, Boston, Massachusetts. 1978.

Russell, A.T., Cantwell, D.P., Mattison, R., and Will, L. A comparison of DSM-II and DSM-III in the diagnosis of childhood psychiatric disorders, III: Multiaxial features. *Archives of General Psychiatry* 1979, *36*:1223–1226.

Schneider, D.M. *American Kinship: A Cultural Account.* Englewood Cliffs, New Jersey: Prentice-Hall, 1968.

Shaffer, D., et al. Early soft neurological signs and later psychopathological development. Read at the annual meeting of the Society for Life History Research in Psychopathology and Society for the Study of Social Biology, New York, New York. November, 1979.

Shaw, C.R., and McKay, H.D. *Juvenile Delinquency and Urban Areas* (rev. ed.). Chicago: University of Chicago Press, 1969.

Spitzer, R.L., Williams, J.B.W., and Skodol, A.E. DSM-III: The major achievements and an overview. *American Journal of Psychiatry* 1980, *137*:151–164.

Suttles, G.D. *The Social Construction of Communities.* Chicago: University of Chicago Press, 1972.

Thoits, P. and Hannan, M. Income and psychological distress: the impact of income-maintenance experiment. *Journal of Health and Social Behavior* 1979, *20*:120–138.

Trussell, T.J. Economic consequences of teenage childbearing. *Family Planning Perspective* 1976, *8*:184–190.

Warren, R.L. *The Community in America.* Chicago: Rand McNally, 1963.

Watt, N.F. Patterns of childhood social development in adult schizophrenics. *Archives of General Psychiatry* 1978, *35*:160–170.

Weissman, M.M., Myers, J.K., Thompson, W.D., Belanger, A. Depressive symptoms as a risk factor for a subsequent first episode of an affective disorder. Read at the Society for Life History Research in Psychopathology and Society for the Study of Social Biology, New York, New York. November, 1979.

Wright, B.D. Solving measurement problems with the Rasch model. *Journal of Educational Measurement* 1977 *14*:97–116.

Studying Children Epidemiologically An International Perspective

TAHA BAASHER, F.R.C. (Psych.)

While child psychiatry has a short history in industrialized countries, its practice in the majority of developing countries is still rather rudimentary and far from being well established. Until two decades ago the social and health concern regarding mental illness was primarily geared toward adult psychiatry and custodial care. Consequently, the sources of information were mainly drawn from statistical reports from mental hospitals and from special institutions for the care of the mentally abnormal offenders. It is therefore not surprising that information about child psychiatric disorders has been generally scarce and often unavailable.

During my experience in Sudan, children were generally brought for psychiatric consultation because of serious mental suffering, mainly psychotic disturbances, mental retardation with physical complications, epilepsy, hysterical conversion, and severe psychoneurotic reactions. Though those below the age of 15 years constituted 45% of the general population, it was estimated that children of this age group who reported with mental disorders formed 10% of the total attendance of psychiatric outpatients. It was clear, however, from general observations that the size of child mental health problems was far greater than what the statistical returns of psychiatric outpatients showed.

The general lack of information about the nature and extent of children with emotional and behavioral disorders in the community, and the keenness to plan relevant and practical facilities to meet the felt needs, prompted us in 1968 to conduct studies among a rural population (Baasher, 1976; Cederblad, 1968). Obviously, there were a number of constraints. Besides the limitation of local resources, field studies in child psychiatry were beset by many difficulties. There were problems of concepts, definitions, sampling, measurement techniques, and a host of epidemiologic questions which had to be answered. These difficulties had to be conceived of within the context of historical perspective, when epidemiologic studies in child psychiatry were generally rare and research methodologies were still in their early stages of development.

This monograph on epidemiologic methods for research in child psychiatry, which provides a general review on the subject and includes useful cross-national material on more recent studies, is therefore timely and important. It is timely for it forms a resourceful reference which should be helpful in the development of better strategies for dealing more effectively with emotional and behavioral problems of children. As rightly stated by Dr. Earls, it is of cardinal importance to take into consideration the overriding issue of how to adapt epidemiologic theories and methods to the situation in developing countries. Some of the studies which were undertaken in more technically advanced countries, such as the parent-teachers' questionnaire, would be inappropriate in certain situations in developing countries and would by necessity have to undergo major adaptation before they could be usefully applied. Because of the well-known inherent constraints, the research procedure may have to be limited to a few items, and the methodological technique has to be relevant to the sociocultural setting. In countries where the illiteracy rate is relatively high, self-reporting or paper-and-pencil methods, for example, may seem out of place, and should therefore not be considered. Again, many of the mental testing methods, including the so-called culture-free tests, may not be suitable in certain situations in developing countries.

Alternatively, simpler testing instruments and more appropriate techniques have to be developed. Such instruments must be subjected to proper assessment and evaluation and should merit the necessary scientific credibility. Moreover, due consideration has to be given to the validity and reliability of such measuring techniques.

Such instruments will naturally assume more importance in comparative research and cross-national studies. In this respect the chapter by Dr. Lotter on Methodological Problems in Cross-Cultural Epidemiologic Research is a worthy effort. Dr. Lotter's findings on childhood autism in Africa is certainly interesting and should stimulate further studies. The methodological difficulties which he clearly indicated are understandable, and several of the issues raised could be resolved through more systematic collaborative work between countries, both technically developed and developing.

Similar to Dr. Lotter's findings, childhood autism has been observed in other parts of Africa, including Sudan. However, for reasons previously stated, there are no reliable statistical data on the incidence of this syndrome nor on its prevalence rate. As generally accepted, there are multiple factors involved in this condition and more studies are needed to unravel the underlying pathogenesis and assess more accurately the psychosocial factors that influence the course of autistic behavior.

It may be relevant to mention here that there are no psychiatric disorders which are commonly known in industrialized countries that do not also occur in developing countries.

However, with improvement in socioeconomic conditions and the better provision of health care, many of the psychosocially disabled children who used to die earlier will have a longer life expectancy and a better chance of being medically diagnosed. More congenital abnormalities and inborn errors of metabolism, for example, have been increasingly spotted. Epiloia (tuberous sclerosis), which was thought previously to be confined to the white race (Brain, 1962) was occasionally seen among indigenous African children. In brief, the presence or absence of certain psychiatric disorders among children in developing countries does not seem at the moment to raise a basic issue. What is more important is the development of action-oriented research studies, within the framework of available resources, for assessing the magnitude of childhood psychiatric disorders and establishing their causative factors. This should be more helpful in setting up the priorities of child mental health problems and in developing ways and means for proper prevention and better management.

In general, the field of childhood psychiatric epidemiology is still riddled with many problems. However, the growing methodology and the increasing scientific interest shown, augur well for future activities and open up new possibilities for epidemiologic studies and better strategies for the extension of child mental health care.

References

Baasher, T.A. Childhood Psychiatric Disorders in the Sudan. *African Journal of Psychiatry,* Vol. 2, No. 1, January 1976.

Brain, R. *Diseases of the Nervous System,* 8th ed. 1977, Oxford University Press.

Cederblad, M. A child psychiatric study on Sudanese Arab Children. *Acta Psychiatrica Scandinavica,* Dec. 4, 1968, Supplement 200, 1–230.

Notes on Contributors

FELTON EARLS, editor of the first volume of our series, is both an epidemiologist and child psychiatrist. His current area of research is the study of the incidence and prevalence of behavioral problems in preschool children and of how childhood psychological problems change as a function of emotional development during the early school years. The research has been based in London, England and in Martha's Vineyard in the United States. Dr. Earls plans to extend his research to other societies in developing countries where nearly three-quarters of the world's children live. He is currently Assistant Professor in Psychiatry at the Harvard Medical School.

THOMAS M. ACHENBACH, a psychologist, is a researcher in the Laboratory of Developmental Psychology at the National Institute of Mental Health in Bethesda, Maryland.

MARGARET E. ENSMINGER, a sociologist, is Assistant Professor of Sociology at Illinois Institute of Technology and Sociologists at the Social Psychiatry Study Center of the University of Chicago.

SHEPPARD G. KELLAM, a psychiatrist, is Professor of Psychiatry and Director of the Social Psychiatry Center at the University of Chicago.

VICTOR LOTTER, a psychologist, is on the faculty of the Department of Psychology at the University of Guelph in Guelph, Ontario in Canada.

HELEN ORVASCHEL, is Assistant Professor of Psychiatry at Yale University where she works in the Depression Research Unit.

NAOMI RICHMAN, a psychiatrist, is Senior Lecturer at the Institute of Child Health in London, England.

LEE N. ROBINS, a sociologist, is Professor of Psychiatry at the Washington University in St. Louis. She will be the editor of the volume in the series entitled Monographs in Psychosocial Epidemiology on drug use studies.

DIANE SHOLOMSKAS is an Associate in Research in the Department of Psychiatry at Yale University and a member of the Research Team in the Depression Research Unit.

MYRNA M. WEISSMAN, an epidemiologist, is Associate Professor of Psychiatry at Yale University and Director of the Depression Research Unit. Together with Dr. Jerome K. Myers, she is coeditor of the volume of the monograph series in psychosocial epidemiology on community surveys.